Play: A Skill for Life

Copyright © 1986 by The American Occupational Therapy Association, Inc.
All rights reserved. No part of this publication may be reproduced, stored in a retrieval system, or transmitted in any form or by any means, electrical, mechanical, photocopying, recording, or otherwise, without the prior written permission of the copyright holder.
Printed in the United States of America.

Library of Congress Catalog Card Number 86-70928

ISBN 0910317-22-4

Cover: Occupational therapist Jean Douglas Clarkson and a student at the Durant-Tuuri-Mott School in Flint, Michigan.

Play
A Skill for Life

A monograph project of the Developmental Disabilities Special Interest Section of the American Occupational Therapy Association

The American Occupational Therapy Association, Inc.
Rockville, Maryland

Contents

Foreword — vii

1.
The Significance of Fostering Play Development in Handicapped Children — 1
Jaime Phillip Muñoz

2.
Evaluating Play Selection And Its Possible Effects on Play Behaviors of Children With Severe Mental Impairment — 13
Sylvia E. Tebo

3.
Play and Therapy, Play or Therapy? — 29
Mechthild Rast

4.
Who Do You Want to Be Today? — 43
The Use of Costumes as Dressing Training in Occupational Therapy
Jean Douglas Clarkson

5.
Infant Play: A Reflection of Cognitive and Motor Development — 55
Diane D'Eugenio

Foreword

The Special Interest Sections of the American Occupational Therapy Association encourage research and publication by their members. This monograph is the second produced by the Developmental Disabilities Special Interest Section (DDSIS), and its focus, play, encompasses issues and information that we hope will find a wide audience among occupational therapy personnel and other health professionals who work with children.

The papers that make up this monograph were chosen from abstracts solicited by a call in the *Occupational Therapy Newspaper* and the *DDSIS Newsletter*. From these abstracts, several authors were invited to submit papers, and it was from these that the final five were selected.

A number of people have contributed to the publication of *Play: A Skill for Life*; most notably, Carol Gwin, OTR, AOTA's liaison to the Special Interest Sections who served as the project's coordinator; Robert Sacheli of AOTA's Publications Division, who edited the manuscript and designed the book's cover and format; and Jaclyn Alexander, Director of Publications, who provided valuable advice and assistance. Linda Tomasini, Practice Division secretary, and Mitchell Cahan, occupational therapy librarian at the American Occupational Therapy Association/Foundation Library, also provided assistance in the publication process.

DDSIS Standing Committee

Charlane Pehoski, MS, OTR, *Coordinating Editor*
Charlotte Exner, MS, OTR
Pat Holtman, OTR
Kathy Swenson Miller, MS, OTR
Lana Warren, MS, OTR

1. The Significance of Fostering Play Development in Handicapped Children

Jaime Phillip Muñoz

Jaime Phillip Muñoz, OTR/L, holds a Bachelor of Science degree in occupational therapy from the University of Kansas. At the Joseph P. Kennedy Memorial Hospital for Children in Brighton, Massachusetts, he handled a varied pediatric caseload including emotionally disturbed, learning disabled, and developmentally disabled children. He currently works at the Boston Veterans Administration Medical Center in Jamaica Plain, Massachusetts.

Fostering Play Development in Handicapped Children

The development of play in children is a subject about which most adults rarely reflect. Play is simply felt to be something that children everywhere know how to do, an act that comes naturally to all. Any parent, however, is acutely aware of how an ailment such as measles, a prolonged fever, or a broken bone may seriously curtail a child's activity level and play. How much more, then, is the play of a child with a congenital or developmental, sensory, intellectual, or physical handicap affected? Play experiences will continue to take a primary role in the early development of such children, but the developmental sequence itself is usually altered and milestones of achievement are more slowly reached. The degree to which an individual child's play is affected by disability depends on that child's own personality as well as the functional limitations of the specific handicaps. Thus, it may not only be the ability to explore and manipulate the environment that may be compromised in a disabled child, but also the ability to experience play in itself. As a result, the handicapped child needs responsible adults to help facilitate the sensory, perceptual, and cognitive stimulation necessary for him or her to learn about and master the environment—one of the important functions of play.

Play and the Handicapped Child

Play has been recognized as a phenomenon that affects physical, emotional, social, and cognitive development. Thus, as a function of childhood, play is seen as essential in facilitating growth in cognitive abilities (1–4) and social development (5–8). What, then, are the specific effects of a congenital or developmental, sensory, intellectual, or physical disability on the play of a child with a handicap?

Mogford (9) states that regardless of the type or extent of the handicap, "all handicapped children have one thing in common—that their ability to explore, interact with, and master the environment is impaired, with a consequent distortion or deprivation of normal childhood experience" (p. 171). Michelman (10) cites some of the common behavioral and learning problems encountered in the handicapped child. These include:

temper tantrums and disruptive behavior, fearfulness of change, inward-directed emotional existence, impaired capacity to confront reality, decreased concentration span, susceptibility to overstimulation, lack of motivation, poor frustration tolerance and fear of failure, poor coordination, inadequate use of language, inability to deal with abstract ideas and feelings of worthlessness and insecurity. (pp. 159–160)

Takata (11) interviewed parents and compiled information that suggests that not only a handicap in itself makes a child's play deficient, but also a play environment that reflects "conditions of play deprivation" (p. 283). Characteristics of such play deprivation include an excess of sedentary activity and television, a lack of raw materials and appropriate models for play, inappropriately high or low parental expectations, and an overemphasis on motor activity rather than the process of exploration and interaction with a toy or the environment (p. 283).

The limitations a handicap places on a child's play behavior are apparent, yet a handicapped child certainly does not lack play. Does the play of the handicapped child differ from that of the nonhandicapped child? If so, how? Are there quantitative and qualitative differences in their play habits? Do handicapped children play spontaneously? Can they be taught to play on developmentally higher levels? In the past 25 years, researchers have increasingly sought to compare the play behavior of normal and handicapped children to answer such questions. Although the outcomes of research are mixed, definite trends have been established.

Tizard (12), for example, found that in a structured, nurturing environment mentally retarded children play at a level commensurate with their mental age. Hulme and Luzner (13) asserted that noninstitutionalized mentally retarded children play spontaneously in a setting that encourages free play. Gregory (14) and Mogford (9) both reported few marked differences in the imaginative play of deaf children compared to their non–hearing-impaired peers. Gregory (14) noted, however, that the play of deaf children is predominantly solitary in nature and delays in imaginative play are seen as such children grow older, possibly due to a lack of development in speech and language that in turn restricts play. Lovell and colleagues (15) compared the play of 3- and 4-year-old language-delayed children to their normal speaking peers and found no significant differences in the amount of time spent on play, the organization of their play, or cooperation. They concluded, however, that for the older children in the group, language served to structure and organize play. They also suggested that speech retardation may affect the intellectual growth of a maturing child.

Research that focuses on deficits in the handicapped child's ability to play is abundant. Lerner, Mardel-Czudnowski, and Goldenberg (16) contended that handicapped children, particularly those with severe handicaps, do not engage in spontaneous play. Wehman (17) asserted that "severely and profoundly retarded persons rarely act on play materials in any constructive manner without some form of external cue, supervision or instruction" (p. 11).

Many writers concur and have documented the failure of retarded children to play spontaneously (18–20). Horne and Philleo (21) found that retarded children preferred more structured play materials and required visual models to engage in constructive play. Fraiberg and Adelson (22) suggested that blind children have similar difficulties and that they require assistance to play. Hewett (23) stated that the spontaneous play of children with cerebral palsy is deficient and suggests that cognitive liabilities may play a more decisive role than physical limitations in the development of play behaviors. Gralewicz's (24) study of play differences between normal and multihandicapped children concluded that the multihandicapped child not only played less, but also had less interactive playtime than the nonhandicapped children.

Mogford (9), based on her experience in running the Toy Library at Nottingham University, discussed some of the difficulties and abnormalities of the play of handicapped children. They include "a lack of sustained attention and rough, destructive and inappropriate use of objects ... persistence of narrow and inflexible methods of exploration ... marked lack of initiative, playing only when encouraged or prompted by an adult" (p. 174). Sheridan (25) commented that disabled children generally learn more slowly and tend to learn basic skills that can be developed only to a very elementary level. She asserts that in order to progress they need "prolonged, patient, individual step-by-step instruction and must be stimulated to constant practice" (p. 118), and a number of authors concur with this summation (9, 10, 11, 17, 26).

The Effects of Structured Play

A number of studies have demonstrated that a structured play environment staffed by trained adults can elicit qualitative and quantitative improvements in a handicapped child's cognitive and social functioning. For instance, Newcomer and Morrison (27) found that institutionalized mentally retarded children who were involved in a systematic developmental play repertoire were found to increase their scores in fine motor, social, and language categories on the Denver Developmental Screening Test. Knapczyk and Yoppi (28) demonstrated that young educable mentally retarded children could be taught to produce and maintain cooperative and competitive play responses when social praise, feedback, and token reward procedures were used. They also suggested that if social play is indeed developmentally hierarchical, as some researchers have suggested (29–31), it then "seems reasonable to assume that by providing reinforcement for specific types of behavior, along with appropriate directions and models of these kinds of behaviors, one might be able to provide for a more rapid movement through the hierarchy" (28, p. 254).

Luria and Yudovitch's (32) classic study of 5-year-old identical twins with limited receptive and expressive language abilities describes the initial primitive play patterns and the development of play activities with intervention and corresponding improvements in language abilities. Wehman (17) reported a study in which retarded adults and adolescents who demonstrated deficits in the quality and quantity of play behaviors were engaged in play activities and taught appropriate use of play materials. After intervention, not only did the clients demonstrate an increase in the type and level of their spontaneous play, but they also required less supervision and direction and were more positive and cooperative during free play.

==Modeling by both adults and normal peers has proved effective in developing play skills in developmentally disabled children.== Peck (33) and colleagues found that such children could be trained and reinforced to imitate the free play of normal children at a similar developmental level. Several authors suggest the importance of imitation as a factor in the development of social and cognitive skills in normal children (8, 34–37).

Occupational Therapy and the Family With a Handicapped Child

The literature that describes the actual practice of occupational therapists working with families of handicapped children is limited. Sparling (38) emphasized that both the handicapped child and parents "may be considered an accessory" or assume a dependent role themselves (p. 7). Tyler and Kogan (39) addressed the quality of interaction between parent and child and suggest that the occupational therapist's role is to "guide the parent of a child with deficits in being an attentive audience and enjoying their child's play" (p. 151). They utilized a series of behavioral instructional programs that focused on mother-child interactions. Mothers were instructed individually, then were given the opportunity to follow the therapists' suggestions with their child in a playroom. They received immediate positive feedback and behavioral instructions through a small device worn in the ear. The results of the study suggest that a reduction in stressful and conflicted interactions is possible through a program of personalized behavioral instruction.

McKibbon (40) described a number of avenues through which a family may be involved in their retarded child's developmental progress. These included classroom volunteer programs, family days, group meetings, and individually prescribed parent training programs for home follow-ups. McKibbon asserted that the occupational therapist can be pivotal in interpreting the results of evaluations to the parents and in outlining home treatment programs. She cautioned that care must be taken to determine whether parents have the emotional and intellectual abilities to carry out programs with their handicapped child or understand the rehabilitation process.

Zisserman (41) notes that parents who come from small nuclear families may lack childrearing experience. She states that "the therapist working with such parents should never assume that the parents possess adequate knowledge about normal child development as a basis for assessing and facilitating their handicapped child's progress" (p. 17). Helping parents to learn about the normal sequence of development and the functional implications of their child's handicap on that sequence can serve to increase their skills and confidence. Zisserman also stressed that therapists should make special efforts to involve fathers in the treatment process by offering evening hours, by organizing "fathers' days," and through well-written home programs.

Crowe (42) agreed on both the importance of family involvement and the necessity of including fathers in treatment programs. He stated that "the involvement of the parents as partners in the enterprise provides an ongoing system which can reinforce the effects of the program while it is in operation, and helps to sustain them after the program's end" (p. 39). He concludes that intentionally or unintentionally excluding half of the parental partnership may be a major barrier in creating an optimal therapeutic environment for the handicapped child.

Individual, group, and home activity programs are the methods of parent intervention most frequently used by occupational therapists. According to Anderson and Hinojosa (43), "potential contact with parents can be significant in occupational therapy because of the needs of many handicapped children for ongoing services" (p. 155). Whenever possible, parents should be guided to discover options on their own and implement the best solutions for their child. Many parents desire a more active role that helps them to develop a sense of mastery and control, and an occupational therapist can facilitate such parental learning.

Friedman's (44) pilot study with parents of children with sensory integrative dysfunction suggested that a parental education program can be effective in promoting an understanding of specific problems and increase the ability to relate constructively to a handicapped child.

A Case for Toys

Michelman (10) underscored the critical need of the handicapped child for therapeutically structured play activities:

> Play is a critical part of the deficit child's treatment with vital influence on his behavior, thinking and performance. No other activity that we know of enables handicapped children to acquire a similar sense of control over their world. If play is to serve the growth needs of the deficit child, it requires continuous structuring and skillful enrichment of the environment.

It is the occupational therapist's role to provide the specific structural and enrichment activities Michelman suggests, based on a knowledge of normal development and the individual child's current perceptual, cognitive, and social functioning. In addition, the therapist should guide parents by offering information, encouragement, and practical measures to make communication with their child more rewarding. Mogford (9) cited the methods used with parents at the Nottingham University Toy Library that include "observation of parents playing with their children, discussion of the child's play, discussion of the play opportunities presented by the toy, and the special adaptations required for individual children" (p. 181). The focus of this approach is not on what a child *cannot* do or *should* be able to do, but what he or she *can* and *is* doing and how parents can interact with a child to enrich these experiences. By identifying a child's level of play and the specific play opportunities presented by toys, the occupational therapist can assist parents in learning about the types of toys to offer and how best to present them.

Dunn and Wodding (45) reported that the length of time a child spends attending to an activity was significantly increased if both the mother and child were focused on the object of the child's play. Sutton-Smith (46) cited Aldrich and Marshall and stated that

It has been found that the greatest increases in response level are recorded for those objects with which the subjects can do most things, that is, which can be handled, moved, seen, touched, and so forth. Further, exploratory and play behavior, like other response systems, is susceptible to increase or diminution in response level as a result of appropriate parental reinforcements (p. 167).

McConkey and associates (47) cited positive results on the use of an instructional video course to aid parents in developing the play behaviors of mentally handicapped children. They sought to inform parents about the developmental stages of play, illustrate techniques for playing with their children, and provide guidelines on how to select, build, and modify toys and activities. Their approach was similar to that advocated by Mogford (48) and Snyder and McLean (49), who focused on the natural interactions of parents and children and identified means by which they could be optimized. Hewett (23), Shere and Kastenbaum (50), Mogford (47), and Sandler and Willis (51) all suggested that parents may need guidance and explicit instruction to select appropriate play activities for their handicapped child.

Research emphasizes the need for and positive outcomes of parents' interacting with their handicapped children. Occupational therapists can promote such interaction through services based on their knowledge of normal patterns of physical, cognitive, and social growth and their understanding of the limitations of specific handicapping situations. Education programs such as that described by McConkey (48), which seek to optimize the parents' natural interactions through play, should be developed. Toy libraries similar to those described by Mogford (9), Junker (52), Riddick (53), and Lear (54) are another means by which toys can be made available and parents can be encouraged to play adaptively with their children. (An appendix to this chapter lists books that can be helpful to both therapists and parents in learning more about the special problems that handicapped children face in play and about means of addressing these needs, particularly through the use of toys.)

Conclusion

Research supports the position that play is a natural learning process that affects all children's physical, cognitive, perceptual, and social development. Play is developmental in nature and, as such, should be encouraged and facilitated. Since the development of play in handicapped children occurs less spontaneously and at a slower rate than that of normal children, occupational therapists need to work with families of such children specifically in the areas of play development or play dysfunction. Often, however, the focus of therapists' concerns have been on the gains in the areas of strengthening perceptual, cognitive, or functional skills. This emphasis can lead to an intrusion on the parenting role, and render parental efforts more frustrating and less rewarding than ideally possible.

Occupational therapists who have familiarized themselves with the developmental sequence of play behaviors can use their knowledge of normal physical, perceptual, cognitive, and social development to work with parents of handicapped children in developing their child's play behaviors. Play presents a naturally occurring, readily structurable activity through which therapists can provide knowledgeable and skillful intervention that can ultimately facilitate a child's growth in a number of important developmental areas.

A logical step in this direction would be for occupational therapists to support the development and existence of toy lending libraries. Here parents can learn what toys are appropriate for their child and how these may be presented, and by the mere provision of such a service and environmental setting, the importance and relevance of play is recognized, supported, and reinforced.

References

1. Fein GG: Pretend play in childhood: An integrative review. *Child Development* 52:1095–1118, 1981
2. Ghiaci G, Richardson JT: The effects of dramatic play upon cognitive development and structure. *J Genetic Psych* 136:77–83, 1980
3. Vandenberg B: Play and development from an ethological perspective. *Amer Psych* 33:724–738, 1978
4. Sylva K: Play and learning. In *Biology of Play*, B. Tizard, D. Harvey, Editors. Philadelphia: Lippincott, 1977
5. Bruner JS: The nature and uses of immaturity. *Am Psych* 27:687–708, 1972
6. Bruner JS, Jolly A, Sylva K (Editors): *Play: Its Role in Development and Evolution*. New York: Basic Books, 1976
7. Guralnick MJ: The social behavior of preschool children at different development levels: Effects of group composition. *J Exper Child Psych* 31:115–130, 1981
8. Piaget J: *Play, Dreams and Imitation in Childhood*. New York: Norton, 1962
9. Mogford K: The play of handicapped children. In *Biology of Play*, B. Tizard, D. Harvey, Editors. Philadelphia: Lippincott, 1977
10. Michelman JS: Play and the deficit child. In *Play as Exploratory Learning*, M. Reilly, Editor. Beverly Hills: Sage Publications, 1974
11. Takata N: The play milieu—A preliminary appraisal. *Am J Occup Ther* 25(6):281–284, 1971
12. Tizard J: *Community Services for the Mentally Handicapped*. Oxford: Oxford University Press, 1964
13. Hulme I, Luzner EA: Play, language and reasoning in subnormal children. *J Child Psychol & Psychiatr* 7:107, 1966

14. Gregory H: *The Deaf Child and His Family*. London: Allen & Unwin, 1976
15. Lovell K, Hoyle HW, Siddall MQ: A study of some aspects of the play and language of young children with delayed speech. *J Child Psychol & Psychiatr* 9:41–50, 1968
16. Lerner J, Mardell-Czudnowski C, Goldenberg D: *Special Education for the Early Childhood Years*. Englewood Cliffs, NJ: Prentice-Hall, 1981
17. Wehman P: *Helping the Mentally Retarded Acquire Play Skills*. Springfield, IL: Charles C Thomas Publishers, 1977
18. Hillman WA, Jr: Therapeutic recreation with the profoundly retarded. *Recreation for the Ill and Handicapped*. Tuscaloosa, AL: National Association of Recreational Therapists, 1967
19. Paloutzian RF, Hasazi J, Streifel J, Edgar C: Promotion of positive social interaction in severely retarded young children. *Am J Mental Deficiency* 75:519–524, 1971
20. Oswin M: *The Empty Hours*. London: Allen Lane, The Penguin Press, 1971
21. Horne B, Philleo C: A comparative study of the spontaneous play activities of normal and mentally defective children. *J Genetic Psych*, 61:33–46, 1942
22. Fraiberg S, Adelson E: Self-representation in language and play: Observations of blind children. *Psychoanalytic Quarterly* 42:539 1973
23. Hewett S: *The Family and the Handicapped Child*. London: Allen & Unwin, 1970
24. Gralewicz A: Play deprivation in multihandicapped children. *Am J Occup Ther* 27(2):70–72, 1973
25. Sheridan M: The importance of spontaneous play in the fundamental learning of handicapped children. *Child Care, Health and Development* 1:3, 1975
26. Li AKF: Play and the mentally retarded child. *Mental Retardation* 19:121–126, 1981
27. Newcomer BL, Morrison TL: Play therapy with institutionalized mentally retarded children. *Am J Mental Deficiency* 78:727–733, 1974
28. Knapczyk DR, Yoppi JO: Development of cooperative and competitive play responses in developmentally disabled children. *Am J Mental Deficiency* 80(3):245–255, 1975
29. Gesell A: *The First Five Years of Life*. New York: Harper & Row 1940
30. Parten MB: Social participation among preschool children. *J Abnormal Psych* 27:243–269, 1932
31. Mueller E, Brenner J: The origins of social skills and interaction among play group toddlers. *Child Development*, 48:854–861, 1977
32. Luria AR, Yudovich F: *Speech and the Development of Mental Processes in the Child*. London: Staples Press, 1959
33. Peck CA, Cooke TP, Apolloni T, Raver S: Teaching retarded preschoolers to imitate free play behavior of non-retarded classmates: Trained and generalized effects. *J Special Ed* 12:195–207, 1978
34. McCall RB, Parke RD, Kavanough RD: Imitation of live and televised models by children one to three years of age. *Monographs of the Society for Research in Child Development*, 42(5), Serial No. 173, 1977
35. Bandura A, Huston AC: Identification as a process of incidental learning. *J Abnormal Psych* 63:311–318, 1961

36. Bandura A, Ross D, Ross SA: Vicarious reinforcement and imitative learning. *J Abnormal Soc Psych* 67:601–607, 1963
37. Bandura A, Huston AC: Identification as a process of incidental learning. In *Early Childhood Play*, M. Almy, Editor. New York: Simon & Schuster, 1968
38. Sparling JW: The transdisciplinary approach with the developmentally delayed child. *Physical and Occupational Therapy in Pediatrics* 1(2):3–13, 1981
39. Tyler NB, Kogan KC: Reduction of stress between mothers and their handicapped children. *Am J Occup Ther* 31(3):151–155, 1977
40. McKibbon EH: An interdisciplinary program for retarded children and their families. *Am J Occup Ther* 26(3):125–129, 1972
41. Zisserman L: The modern family and rehabilitation of the handicapped: A macrosociological view. *Am J Occup Ther* 35(1):13–20, 1981
42. Crowe TK: Father involvement in early intervention programs. *Physical and Occupational Therapy in Pediatrics* 1(3):35–46, 1981
43. Anderson J, Hinojosa J: Parents and therapists in a professional partnership. *Am J Occup Ther* 38(7):452–461, 1984
44. Friedman B: A program for parents of children with sensory integrative dysfunction. *Am J Occup Ther* 36(9):586–589, 1982
45. Dunn J, Wooding C: Play in the home and its implications for learning. In *Biology of Play*, B. Tizard, D. Harvey, Editors. Philadelphia: Lippincott, 1977
46. Sutton-Smith B: The role of play in cognitive development. In *Early Childhood Play*, M Almy, Editor. New York: Simon & Schuster, 1967
47. McConkey R, McEvoy J, Gallagher F: Learning through play: The evaluation of a video course for parents of mentally handicapped children. *Child Care Health and Development* 8:348–359, 1982
48. Mogford K: Developing the play of young mentally handicapped children through the participation of parents. *Research Exchange and Practice in Mental Retardation* 2:40–46, 1976
49. Snyder LK, McLean JE: Deficient acquisition strategies: A proposed framework for analyzing severe language deficiency. *Am J Mental Deficiency* 81:288–299, 1977
50. Shere E, Kastenbaum R: Mother-child interactions and cerebral palsy. Environmental and psychosocial obstacles to cognitive development. *Genetic Psychology Monographs* 73(2), 1966
51. Sandler A, Willis DM: Preliminary notes on play and mastery in the blind child. *J Child Psych* 1(3):7, 1965
52. Junker KS: A center for play habilitation as an indispensable part of the medical and educational care of handicapped and sick children. *Pediatrician* 3:315, 1974
53. Riddick B: *Toys and Play for the Young Handicapped Child*. London: Croom Helm, 1982
54. Lear R: *Play Helps: Toys and Activities for Handicapped Children*. London: Heinemann Health Books, 1977

Appendix
Resources on Play and the Child with a Handicap

The Family and the Handicapped Child—A Study of Cerebral Palsied Children in their Homes—Sheila Hewett with John and Elizabeth Newson, 1970, Chicago: Aldine Publishing

Reports research on the practical problems that mothers of handicapped children face in daily care and their evaluation of the efficacy of available social services. Compares characteristics of the family life of normal and handicapped children.

Toys, Play and Discipline in Childhood—Beatrix Tudor-Hart, 1955, London: Routledge and Kegan, Paul

Explores the link between play and discipline and suggests that play provides the social arena in which self-discipline is learned. Emphasizes the parental importance of both a knowledge of play development and the careful provision of appropriate play materials as a means of facilitating social growth.

Toys and Play Things: In Development and Remediation—John and Elizabeth Newton, 1979, New York: Pantheon Books

An excellent book that discusses many facets of play including its normal development, stages, and types; the importance of toys in facilitating the developmental progression; and the use of toys for specific therapeutic aims. Provides a rich resource list that indexes research in various areas of play development and toy use.

Handling the Young Cerebral Palsied Child at Home—Nancie Finnie, 1975, New York: Dutton

A practical guide for parents that offers advice on play activities for severely handicapped children.

Helping the Mentally Retarded Acquire Play Skills—Paul Wehman, 1977, Springfield, IL: Charles C Thomas Publishers

Offers guidelines for developing play programs for severely or profoundly retarded children. Reviews literature and research findings on the play development of normal and mentally retarded children.

You Can Raise Your Handicapped Child—Evelyn West Ayrault, 1964, New York: Putnam

An encouraging guide for parents of handicapped children that provides practical information on the nature of and intervention for social, cognitive, and behavioral deficits. Provides lists of appropriate toys, guidelines on their selection, and recommendations on the type of toys suitable for different age groups and specific therapeutic aims.

Toys and Play for the Young Handicapped Child—Barbara Riddick, 1982, London: Croom Helm

Offers enlightened details and descriptions about the role of toys and play for both normal and handicapped children. Offers thorough toy lists and suggestions for their use with handicapped children. Outlines important skills in the development of children from infancy to nursery school age.

Play Helps: Toys and Activities for Handicapped Children—Roma Lear, 1977, London: Heinemann Health Books

Written primarily as an idea book for parents that will facilitate new playtime activities, emphasizing those that can be integrated into the routines of daily living. Categorizes play ideas according to the specific sense that each is designed to stimulate.

2. Evaluating Toy Selection

And Its Possible Effects on Play Behaviors of Children With Severe Mental Impairment

Sylvia E. Tebo

Sylvia E. Tebo, MS, OTR, is a staff occupational therapist at Total Therapy Management's Cognitive Restructuring Center in Flint, Michigan. This pilot study was completed in partial fulfillment of the requirements for a Master of Science degree in occupational therapy at Western Michigan University, Kalamazoo, Michigan.

Evaluating Toy Selection

According to Takata (1), "Play provides for the child's advancement to new stages of mastery, play for the adult provides sideward stepping into another reality" (p. 281). Play on the part of children involves their discovery of the world and themselves; the equivalent discovery of the world and people by adults is called science. Play, therefore, is very serious work.

Without play, a developing child would not progress beyond 5 months of age, when the motor ability to reach out and to bring the hands together to explore the environment and self is developed (2). Play has been variously described as neuromuscular, sensory, mental, social, spontaneous, and pleasurable (1, 3, 4). Play has been equated with the practice of adult roles, cognitive development, use of surplus energy, revitalization of the mental and physical being, recapitulation of the phylogenetic process, reduction of tension, and development of competence (1, 5–8). Slobin (9) summarized play most succinctly by commenting that "when we observe play, we find ourselves faced with hundreds of years of attempts to understand human behavior" (p. 59).

The majority of play literature has been based on normal populations. Lack of research on toys for and play behaviors of severely handicapped children has warranted further investigation of their toy play behaviors and of appropriate prescription of toys for this population. This chapter focuses on a research study in which toys most frequently used in selected school programs for severely mentally impaired children in Michigan were reviewed. The research was designed to increase the knowledge and resources in the area of toy play and related behaviors and to document the need for careful selection of toys for this population.

Review of Related Literature

The Importance of Play in Normal and Abnormal Development

The importance of play in development has been stressed by Piaget (10), Reilly (11), and Florey (12). Play ranks with eating and sleeping in importance as an influence on development (10, 11, 13). While much research has been done in the area of play behavior of normal children, little has been done to support the generalization of these findings to the handicapped population, especially children with multiple handicaps.

Normal children acquire information about their world through experimentation with and observation of events around them. Wehman and Abrahamson (6) stated that handicapped children often lack the necessary skills of attending, persistence, and discrimination to learn as normal children do through experimentation and observation. The learning process is even more difficult for children with physical handicaps.

A study done by Weiner, Tilton, and Ottinger (14) reevaluated their previous work (15) comparing toy play behaviors of autistic, retarded, and normal children who were all without physical handicaps. The use of toys was recorded on 10 predetermined, operationally defined categories of play.

A significant difference was found among the three groups of children. Normal children showed a larger repertoire of play behaviors than retarded children, and both of these groups were higher in this area than the autistic children. Autistic children showed a higher number of repetitive acts, and the retarded children showed a higher number of undefined uses over the other groups.

Weiner and Weiner (16) also compared toy play behaviors of normal and retarded children without physical handicaps. The researchers' aim was to develop an appropriate cognitive evaluation for retarded children. The retarded children were matched with normal 3- and 6-year-olds by maturational age (MA) and chronological age, respectively.

Toy play behaviors observed were: combinational use, separation of parts, personalized use, pushing or pulling, throwing, pounding, oral contact, repetitive manual manipulation, and undefined use. The retarded children showed more oral contact, repetitive manual manipulation, and undefined use than did the two groups of normal 6- and 3-year-olds. (Differences were noted between the normal 6-year-olds and the normal 3-year-olds, but they are not pertinent to this discussion.)

The intent of the researchers in both studies (14, 16) was to develop a method of more accurately diagnosing children for special education programs. The studies also provide valuable documentation to support two key issues: (a) because the play behaviors of normal and handicapped children are significantly different, results of research in play behavior of normal children are not easily generalized to handicapped populations; and (b) more research is justified and needed to document the toy play behaviors of all handicapped children.

Influence of the Environment on Play

Nonhuman Environment. Some research has been done specifically on the play behavior of severely retarded children with toys as a part of the environment. Toy play in severely retarded children has been observed in terms of visual exploration, grasping, crawling, walking, attention, language, exploration, manipulation, and socialization (12). Toys were considered as a significant part of a total environment in which a child must develop and grow (17, 18). Hutt and Hutt (19), Davenport and Berkson (20), and Berkson and Mason (21) found that the environment that included toys (as opposed to those without toys) could be arranged to reduce maladaptive behaviors and to reinforce desired behaviors by including toys that children preferred.

Human Environment. Another important part of the environment is the presence of positive reinforcement and role models for appropriate toy play behaviors. Florey (12) included imitation of role models as a part of the conditions to facilitate play.

Wehman and Marchant (22) found that through modeling, instruction, and verbal reinforcement, four severely retarded 6-year-olds improved their independent and social play skills. The researchers' premise was that free play skills, defined as "any action or combination of actions with objects the child engages in for the apparent purpose of fun" (p. 110), influenced the development of social, cognitive, and language skills. The definition of play, which could have been any action that was not destructive, allowed for a wide range of behaviors, including repetitive and nonpurposeful behaviors.

Hopper and Wambold (23) reported on the documentation of "instructional procedures" to increase independent play in severely mentally impaired children. The researchers' premise was that children who could play independently would allow teachers to devote more time to other classroom activities. Independent play would also assist the child's return to a home living situation because it would allow increased respite time for care givers. Toys were classified as reactive (producing movement or tactile or auditory feedback when acted on) or nonreactive (requiring representational or imaginative play that limited feedback). The researchers were interested in determining whether reactive toys would increase independent play more or less than nonreactive toys as teachers were systematically phased from the free play environment. The researchers found no preference for either type of toy, and it was suggested that faulty sampling techniques or the nature of the toys available for observation might be sources of error. The authors' interpretation of the results suggested that some children with severe mental impairment might have played independently if they had been given a variety of developmentally appropriate toys. No analysis was done to substantiate this assertion. The only results given were percentages of inappropriate or appropriate play, and the only accurate conclusions drawn from toy interactions was that the children showed no preference for reactive or nonreactive toys and that there was no significant difference in the children's behavior with reactive or nonreactive toys.

Evaluation and Selection of Toys for Handicapped Children

As a result of the research on teaching methods and toy play behavior, researchers have attempted to classify and evaluate the effectiveness of toys used with the handicapped population, expressing a concern for providing interesting and stimulating toys for severely impaired children. Because children who are severely impaired have a limited ability to engage in symbolic activity, their toys should be novel, diverse, immediately reinforcing, and commensurate with the child's individual mental age and functional level (3, 24).

Watters and Wood (25) assessed the effects of three classes of toys (soft [stuffed], hard, and wheeled) on the play and self-stimulatory behavior of a group of autistic and severely handicapped boys. The toy interactions monitored were: contact, orientation toward the toys, manipulation of the toys, self-stimulation, and motion.

Results were recorded as percentages of occurrence of the type of interaction. For each child, the percentages of contact and manipulation were less for soft toys. A greater percentage (2.38 times) of self-stimulation and motion occurred with soft toys than with hard or wheeled toys. A significant difference between the percentage of contact with hard and soft toys and the percentage of soft and wheeled toys existed; however, no significant difference existed between the percentage of contact with wheeled and hard toys.

This study noted the importance of evaluation and selection of toys along with training in appropriate toy play. The limitations noted were that the children were all male, that they were not in a free play situation, and that they were not allowed to choose the toy.

Flavell and Cannon (24) researched toy preferences among 11 severely mentally impaired females. Appropriate engagement (manipulation, visually attending, listening) with designated toys was recorded. Inappropriate engagements, which were not scored, were stereotypic, dangerous, or destructive behaviors. The results showed that preference for toys did not correlate with the price of the toy and that the professional staff involved was not accurate in predicting which toys the subjects would prefer.

Even though the researchers cautioned against drawing conclusions from this study, results showed that proper toy selection can be effective in improving behavior, since the most popular toys were appropriately used 75% of the time they were available. The study also provided a basis for further research into toy preferences of handicapped people and prescription of toys by professionals. The investigators suggested that future research identify common features of preferred toys, thus making it possible to develop better toys by assembling optimum combinations of features for various subpopulations of handicapped individuals.

Wehman (3), Guthrie (5), and Kesner and Sunal (26) all discussed criteria for selection of toys for children with severe mental impairments. Guthrie (5) looked at development in visually impaired children and developed the following criteria for toy selection. The toy should:

- Fit goals and objectives for the child;
- Account for residual vision;
- Establish skills;
- Provide basic concrete experiences;
- Stimulate the child and promote sensory awareness (auditory, gustatory, olfactory, visual, tactile); and
- Allow manipulation.

The personality and needs of the individual were stressed. This study also emphasized the need for a classification system for toys in special education. Several factors influencing toy purchase were also discussed. The toy's purpose and function should allow:

Evaluating Toy Selection

→ *toy's purpose/function should allow:*
- Establishment of rapport;
- Stimulation of senses;
- Demonstration of the child's skills; and
- Development of skills/concepts.

Factors considered relating to the child's environment should include:

- Cost;
- Use (classroom or home, inside or outside);
- Transportability;
- Versatility;
- Life-style of child and family; and
- Number of parts that could be lost.

Kesner and Sunal (26) presented a "toy evaluation checklist" that rated toys according to 15 criteria representing safety, practicality, price, versatility, educational value, and developmental appropriateness. Their suggested criteria were general enough that specific skills could be defined for any population under the category of developmental appropriateness and thus the checklist could be used with any handicapped population.

Wehman (3) reviewed the literature on toy play and urged researchers to further study the stimulus characteristics of toys so that the findings could be applied to play skill development of children with severe mental impairment. Wehman further noted that toys used in schools at the time of the study failed to evoke play activity in children with severe mental impairment. It is difficult to determine from this study whether the toys themselves or the teachers' toy play teaching styles failed to evoke play activity in the children, since previous research has indicated that play behaviors are learned (14–16).

Summary

This review indicates that the play behavior of developmentally disabled children may be significantly different as compared to normal children (14–16). It would also appear that the appropriate selection of toys for disabled children is important in order to maximize their constructive interaction (3, 5, 26). Thus, it would appear to be important to know what toys are commonly available to a child in a teaching situation. The pilot study reported below is an initial attempt to discover the toys that are commonly available to children in classrooms for the severely mentally impaired.

The Pilot Study

see p. 26

A survey document was developed asking teachers of severely mentally impaired children to list the 10 toys most frequently used (Appendix 1). The teachers were also asked to indicate whether the toys chosen were used for sensory stimulation, behavioral training, or fine motor, gross motor, socialization, or cognitive skill development (see definitions in Appendix

2). The 30 teachers surveyed were all employed by the Michigan Intermediate School District.

Five children from one of the surveyed teacher's classrooms were observed by the examiner as they interacted with the five toys most commonly listed in the survey. Each of the children had been diagnosed as severely mentally impaired and was so listed on his or her individualized education plan according to the Michigan Department of Education Guidelines (27). They had no other handicapping conditions. The children ranged in age from 3 years, 2 months to 9 years, 2 months and had IQs ranging from 30 to 50 (WISC). There were four boys and one girl.

Each child was seen individually in an isolated corner of the classroom during the normal free play time. Observations of the children's toy interactions were entered on an observation record, using an interval recording method. Each toy was presented for 4 minutes, with the child's performance being recorded after each 50-second interval of observation. The children were seen on three separate occasions. The behaviors observed were recorded in one of the following areas: fine motor, gross motor, social skills, cognitive skill, or speech and language. The same definitions used in the teachers' survey were used in the observational record form (Appendix II). For example, a social interaction might include the child's offering a toy to the observer. A gross motor interaction might include throwing a toy or walking away with it. A cognitive interaction might include any purposeful use or meaningful exploratory interaction with the toy. Speech and language indicated any vocalization or language observed.

Results

Of the 30 surveys mailed to teachers of children with severe mental impairments, 16 were returned. Table 1 lists all the toys that were included by the teachers on the survey form. The most commonly listed toys included puzzles (16 entries), balls (13 entries), pegs and pegboards (11 entries), beads and string (8 entries), and blocks (8 entries). Table 1 also summarizes each teacher's response on how these toys were used. Table 2 indicates how the children actually engaged in play with the five most commonly used toys. Of these, four (puzzles, pegs and pegboard, beads and string, blocks) seemed to have a high frequency of use by teachers in the development of fine motor skills. It would also appear that in a free play situation these toys elicited fine motor behavior in severely mentally impaired children.

Another correlation between teacher goals and child interactions is seen in the use of the ball. The ball provided an opportunity for gross motor behavior on the part of the child during free play, in agreement with the goal indicated by the teachers for this toy. The ball also appeared to promote social interaction in the free play situation, although this was not as frequently listed as a use of this toy by the teachers. None of the other toys observed seemed to promote social interaction during free play.

Evaluating Toy Selection

Table 1
Summary of Teacher Survey

			No. Times Behavioral Categories Were Checked							
No. Times Listed	Description	Source	FM	GM	SO	CS	SL	SS	BT	RS
16	Puzzles	Judy Hammett Playskool Kohner Fisher Price Lauri	9	3	0	11	6	4	1	2
13	Balls, ball games	Fisher Price School prods. catalogs	2	8	4	2	3	5	2	6
11	Pegboards, pegs	Tactilmat Hammett	6	0	1	3	0	1	0	0
8	Blocks, building sets	Scrap wood School prods. catalogs	8	5	6	4	5	3	4	4
8	Beads, string	Playskool Ideal School prods. catalogs	6	0	0	3	0	2	0	0
7	Busy Box	Child Guidance Gabriel Fisher Price	7	1		5	4	7	3	4
5	Shape Sorters	Fisher Price Tupperware Hasbro	3			3	1	2		
4	Crayons		4	1	1	2		3	1	2
4	See-n-Say	Mattel	1		1	2	3	2	2	1
3	Rhythm instruments	Child Guid.	2	1	3	1	2	2	2	2
3	Play Doh		3			1	1	3		
3	Stacking rings	Hammett	3	2	1	2	1	2	1	1
3	Tempera paint		2	1	1	1		3	1	2
3	Push-pull toys	Fisher Price	2	2		1	1			1
2	Musical Radio	Michigan Products	1	1			1	1	1	
2	Toy music boxes	Ideal			1		1		1	1

KEY: FM — Fine motor SO — Social skills SL — Speech and language BT — Behavioral training
     GM — Gross motor CS — Cognitive skills SS — Sensory stimulation RS — Recreational skills

Sylvia E. Tebo

2	Scooter boards			11	11			11		
2	Lite Brite	Hasbro	2		1	2		2		
2	Mobiles				1	1	1	1	1	1
2	Bubbles		1	1		1		1		1
2	Dolls		1	1	2	1	1	2	2	1
2	Records, movement	Hap Palmer		2	1	1	2	1	2	2
1	Jack-in-the-Box	Child Guid.	1				1		1	
1	Records, fingerplays	Michigan Prods.	1	1	1	1	1	1		1
1	Little Tooter Trumpet	Tomy				1	1		1	1
1	Magical Musical Thing	Fisher Price	1	1				1		
1	Toy tape player		1		1		1	1	1	
1	Wind-up Musical Train	Tomy	1				1	1	1	
1	Aerobat			1	1	1	1		1	1
1	Fun Tunnel	Discovery Toys		1	1			1		
1	T-Car	Discovery Toys		1	1				1	1
1	Riding Toys	Fisher Price		1						1
1	Rhythm Rollers	Johnson & Johnson	1				1	1		
1	Surprise Box	Child Guid.	1			1				
1	Vibrator						1	1		
1	Family Play House	Fisher Price			1	1	1		1	
1	Preschool Mr. Potato Head				1	1	1		1	
1	Cogwheels and Cranks						1			
1	Poppin' Pals		1			1	1	1		
1	Sesame Street Top			1		1	1	1	1	1
1	Happy Hoppers			1	1			1		1
1	Clackety Truck			1				1		1
1	Puppets		2	1	2	1	2	2	2	1
1	Tinker Toys		1			1		1		
1	Preschool Legos		1		1					1
1	Colored chalk		1	1	1	1		1	1	1

Evaluating Toy Selection

Table 1, continued
Summary of Teacher Survey

No. Times Listed	Description	Source	FM	GM	SO	CS	SL	SS	BT	RS
1	Picture Bingo				1	1	1			
1	Uno Cards				1	1			1	
1	Peabody Pictures Series					1	1			
1	Clear stencils		1							
1	Day-by-day calendar				1	1		1		
1	Brimax board books	Discovery Toys			1	1	1		1	
1	Scissors		1							
1	Picture cards		1			1	1	1		

Interpretation of Survey Results

The teachers surveyed in this pilot study appeared to have a variety of toys available to use with the children in their classrooms. Of interest is the fact that the five toys listed as most often used are nonreactive according to the Hopper and Wambold's (23) definition. Several reactive toys were listed, but with a lower frequency; many of these tended to be rated high in sensory stimulation. No computerized toys or games were listed, even though the use of computers in education is widely expanding.

One of the limitations of this pilot study was the lack of information on the specific part of the school day in which the teachers used the listed toys. It would have been helpful to have

Table 2
Occurrence of Behaviors during Observations Stated in Percentages

	FM	GM	SO	CS	SL
Puzzle	69	22	0	1	8
Ball	30	46	10	3	11
Pegs and pegboard	74	17	0	2	7
Beads and string	59	21	0	8	12
Blocks	65	19	0	7	9

KEY: FM — Fine motor
GM— Gross motor
SO — Social skills
CS — Cognitive skills
SL — Speech and language

known whether the toys were used primarily in one-on-one teaching situations or during free play. In the observation section of this study, it was noted that the observers' noninteraction with the children (observing the child and not actively participating in the child's interaction with the toy) often resulted in the child's noninteraction with the toy. The child might walk away from the toy or simply manipulate small parts (a single block, bead, or puzzle piece). Some interaction could be defined as self-stimulatory. It would, therefore, appear necessary to define toys as being more appropriate for one-on-one learning situations or for non-adult-directed free play.

This distinction between toys used for free play and those used for structured learning rests on which toys will stimulate the child's interaction and which toys require an adult to initiate interaction. Interaction with an adult is necessary to teach some play skills to severely impaired children (21); however, the repeated need for such adult initiation poses questions of the interest value of the toy as well as of the developmental level of play in a given child. What are the characteristics of a toy that elicit nondirected, appropriate interaction by a child with severe mental impairment? Many commercially available toys appear to have the potential to meet the needs of severely impaired children, and many can be adapted to meet the specific needs of an individual child. In addition, the introduction of microswitches and microcomputers has opened a new world for severely impaired children.

As previously noted, children's play involves their discovery of the world and themselves. Play is indeed very serious work. Toys that promote this discovery are important tools in a child's life. More exploration is needed on the subject of appropriate toys and their use with severely impaired children. The occupational therapist with training in human development and activity analysis has the optimal combination of skills to assist teachers in selecting and adapting toys that will best meet a child's specific needs. To better assist in this process, therapists need to know more about how toys are used in the classroom and how handicapped children play with toys.

This pilot study has been a first step in solving this problem. It points to the need to define toys in relation to how they will be used (i.e., as tools for teaching or therapeutic intervention or to promote exploration during free play). It also points out the need for professionals to look at the unique nature of the toy play behavior of severely impaired children.

References

1. Takata N: The play milieu—A preliminary appraisal. *Am J Occup Ther* 25:281–284, 1971
2. Bobath B, Bobath K: *Motor Development in the Different Types of Cerebral Palsy.* London: William Heinemann Medical Books Limited, 1982

3. Wehman P: Selection of play materials for the severely handicapped: A continuing dilemma. *Education and Training of the Mentally Retarded* 11(1):46–50, 1976
4. Florey LL: Studies of play: Implications for growth, development, and for clinical practice. *Am J Occup Ther* 35:519–524, 1981
5. Guthrie S: Criteria for educational toys for pre-school visually impaired children. *Journal of Visual Impairment and Blindness* 17(4):144–146, 1979
6. Wehman P, Abrahamson M: Three theoretical approaches to play: Applications for exceptional children. *Am J Occup Ther* 30:551–559, 1976
7. Mead GH: *Mind, Self and Society*. Chicago: University of Chicago Press, 1934
8. White RW: Motivation reconsidered: The concept of competence. In *Readings in Child Behavior and Development*, 2nd Edition. New York: Harcourt Brace & World, 1964, pp 164–191
9. Slobin I: Fruits of the first season: A discussion of the role of play in childhood. *Journal of Humanistic Psychology* 4(1):59–79, 1964
10. Piaget J: *Play, Dreams, and Imitation in Childhood*. New York: WW Norton, 1962
11. Reilly M (Editor): *Play as Exploratory Learning*. Beverly Hills, CA: Sage Publications, 1974
12. Florey L: An approach to play and play development. *Am J Occup Ther* 25:275–280, 1971
13. Wilkinson PF: *In Celebration of Play*. New York: St. Martin's Press, 1980
14. Weiner BJ, Ottinger DR, Tilton JR: Comparison of the toy-play behavior of autistic, retarded, and normal children: A reanalysis. *Psychol Rep* 25:223–227, 1969
15. Tilton JR, Ottinger DR: Comparison of the toy play behavior of autistic, retarded, and normal children. *Psychol Rep* 15:967–975, 1964
16. Weiner EA, Weiner BJ: Differentiation of retarded and normal children through toy-play analysis. *Multivariate Behavioral Research* 9(2):245–252, 1974
17. Horner RD: The effects of an environmental enrichment program on the behavior of institutionalized profoundly retarded children. *J Appl Behav Anal* 13(3):473–491, 1980
18. Wehman P: Effects of different environmental conditions on leisure time activity of the severely and profoundly handicapped. *Journal of Special Education* 12(2):183–193, 1983
19. Hutt C, Hutt S: Effects of environmental complexity on stereotyped behaviors in children. *Animal Behavior* 13(1):1–4, 1965
20. Davenport R, Berkson B: Stereotyped movements of mental defectives: II. Effects of novel objects. *Am J Ment Defic* 67:879–882, 1963
21. Berkson G, Mason W: Stereotyped movements of mental defectives: IV. The effects of toys and the character of acts. *Am J Ment Defic* 68:511–524, 1964
22. Wehman P, Marchant J: Improving free play skills of severely retarded children. *Am J Occup Ther* 32:100–104, 1978
23. Hopper C, Wambold C: Improving the independent play of severely mentally retarded children. *Education and Training of the Mentally Retarded* 13:42–46, 1978
24. Flavell JE, Cannon PR: Evaluation of entertainment materials for severely retarded persons. *Am J Ment Defic* 81:357–361, 1976

25. Watters RG, Wood DE: Play and self-stimulatory behaviors of autistic and other severely dysfunctional children with different classes of toys. *Journal of Special Education* 17(1):27–35, 1983
26. Kesner JR, Sunal CS: Choosing the right toy: A checklist. *International Journal of Early Childhood* 2(2):76–80, 1980
27. Michigan Department of Education. *Michigan Department of Education Guidelines*. Lansing, MI: Author, 1982

Evaluating Toy Selection

Appendix 1
Teacher Questionnaire

1. List the toys you use most frequently (up to ten):

   Name   Manufacturer/source
   1.
   2.
   3.
   4.
   5.
   6.
   7.
   8.
   9.
   10.

2. Of the preceding toys that you use most frequently, check below the ones used for: (by number)

   Sensory stimulation:
   1__ 2__ 3__ 4__ 5__ 6__ 7__ 8__ 9__ 10__

   Fine motor:
   1__ 2__ 3__ 4__ 5__ 6__ 7__ 8__ 9__ 10__

   Gross motor:
   1__ 2__ 3__ 4__ 5__ 6__ 7__ 8__ 9__ 10__

   Behavioral training:
   1__ 2__ 3__ 4__ 5__ 6__ 7__ 8__ 9__ 10__

   Socialization:
   1__ 2__ 3__ 4__ 5__ 6__ 7__ 8__ 9__ 10__

   Cognitive skills:
   1__ 2__ 3__ 4__ 5__ 6__ 7__ 8__ 9__ 10__

   Recreational skills:
   1__ 2__ 3__ 4__ 5__ 6__ 7__ 8__ 9__ 10__

   Speech and language:
   1__ 2__ 3__ 4__ 5__ 6__ 7__ 8__ 9__ 10__

   Other purposes: (please state)
   1__ 2__ 3__ 4__ 5__ 6__ 7__ 8__ 9__ 10__
   1__ 2__ 3__ 4__ 5__ 6__ 7__ 8__ 9__ 10__

   Comments:

Appendix 2
Questionnaire Category Definitions

Visual stimulation   The toy is used to give a child visual input through color, shape, reflection of light or images, or any combination of these characteristics.

Tactile stimulation   Input is given through touching soft, rough, uneven, unusually textured surfaces or familiar shapes.

Auditory stimulation   The toy is used to give a child input through familiar or new sounds, music, or voices.

Fine motor   The toy is used to reinforce or stimulate any select movements using the fingers of one or both hands to grasp or manipulate any object, or to promote dexterity.

Gross motor   The toy is used to reinforce or stimulate movement involving self-mobility using arms and/or legs, reaching for an object or carrying it while mobile, climbing, rolling, jumping, or throwing.

Behavioral training   The toy is used as a tool to reinforce a behavior or to teach a behavior.

Social skills   The toy is used to facilitate sharing, parallel play, cooperative play, or role playing.

Cognitive skills   The toy is used to reinforce exploring, sequencing, discrimination of size or shape, one-to-one correspondence, symbol recognition, memory, attention, concentration, problem solving, decision making.

Recreational skills   The toy is used to reinforce or to stimulate play for fun or entertainment or to develop skills a child can use in leisure hours.

Speech and language   The toy is used to encourage speech or to develop a child's receptive or expressive language skills.

Definitions were taken from these resources:

Anderson RM, Greer JG (Editors): *Educating the Severely and Profoundly Retarded*. Baltimore: University Park Press, 1980

Hom HL Jr, Robinson PA (Editors): *Psychological Processes in Early Education*. New York: Academic Press, 1977

Wilkinson PF: *In Celebration of Play*. New York: St. Martin's Press, 1980

3. Play and Therapy, Play or Therapy?

Mechthild Rast

Mechthild Rast, MS, OTR *received her diploma in occupational therapy in Zurich, Switzerland. She holds a BA from Antioch University, Seattle, Washington, and a MS in occupational therapy from the University of Washington, Seattle. An occupational therapy instructor in neurodevelopmental treatment courses, she is also certified to administer and interpret the Southern California Sensory Integration Test. She works in private practice in Seattle and lectures internationally.*

Play and Therapy, Play or Therapy?

Play and therapy almost appear to be mutually exclusive. A child's play is an intrinsically motivating activity done voluntarily and for its own sake (1, 2); therapy proceeds according to the therapist's plan to achieve definite treatment objectives. Also, play is characterized by a combination of engagement and enjoyment, characteristics that may be desirable in therapy, but are not necessarily typical of it. With this dichotomy, why do pediatric therapists try to incorporate play into therapy programs? Play offers a practical vehicle to enlist a child's attention, to practice specific motor and functional skills, and to promote sensory processing, perceptual abilities, and cognitive development. It also serves to support social, emotional, and language development. In the therapeutic setting, play often becomes a tool used to work toward a goal, despite the fact that the goal-oriented, externally controlled aspects of the therapy situation conflict with the essence of play itself.

Therefore, a differentiation is suggested between the terms *play* and *play activities*. The therapy setting for the disabled child rarely can incorporate all the essential characteristics of play, but therapy may include activities that incorporate some of its aspects. These play activities can facilitate the achievement of therapy goals, one of which may be the promotion of play development.

This paper relates aspects of normal play development to the clinical assessment and treatment of developmentally disabled children and provides guidelines for selecting and incorporating appropriate play activities into therapy. Disabled children with neuromuscular disorders are the particular focus of its discussion.

Whether play activities are used to facilitate learning or to enhance play development, the knowledge of normal play development must be combined with an awareness of the individual child's abilities, interests, and limitations.

A review of the types of play typical of certain developmental stages relates to the first four of Erikson's "Eight Ages of Man" (3). While Erikson's psychoanalytic interpretations go beyond the scope of this paper, each of his stages entails specific aspects of growth and crisis in the evolving personality, from which implications and practical suggestions for the disabled child can be derived. For example, how might a disability affect normal play development? How can aspects of normal play be used in therapy and how can that therapy contribute to normal play development?

The Sensorimotor Period

The unimpaired infant's sensory systems combined with the developing control of movement contribute to the acquisition of exploratory and play behavior. During the first year of life, infants explore their bodies (4) and the environment. Their relatively crude motor control is used to interact with the environment in repetitive and undifferentiated ways (5). Mouthing, banging, waving, scratching, and throwing are frequently observed behaviors

(6–9). Infants impose their own interaction schemes on an object or toy regardless of its specific purpose. Their behavior, however, is affected by certain attributes of objects. McCall (10) found that the length of time an infant stays involved with an object seems to be influenced by its sound-producing potential and plasticity. Infants are attracted by an object's responsiveness to their movements. By the end of the first year and during the second year, an infant's behavior reveals an increasing understanding of the functional use of familiar objects such as a cup, spoon, or comb. Children relate familiar objects first to their bodies (6–8). Functional use of objects precedes representational play. Around the same time, interest in spatial characteristics and a beginning awareness of shared attributes among objects result in container play, stacking, and grouping (7–9, 11).

The developing motor abilities are an important source of enjoyment. Control against gravity and various means of locomotion allow a child to explore and become familiar with the surrounding space. According to Bruner (12), play during this period provides the opportunity to try out flexible patterns of interaction with the environment that consequently can become part of more complex skills. He emphasizes the importance of self-initiated intentional behavior, sustained attention, and adequate social support.

Additional dimensions to the meaning of the sensorimotor period are suggested by Erikson (3), whose first stage is called "Basic Trust vs. Basic Mistrust." The foundation of trust is a sense of security and predictability. The unimpaired infant's social trust is believed to be enhanced through the ease of feeding. Infants gain trust in their bodies in relation to gravity and the space around them. They experience gradual control over upright positions and sense that, even when falling, their reliable protective reactions offer security. The emergence of object permanence assists in developing a sense of trust in the existence of people and objects that are temporarily out of sight. The evolving sense of security is accompanied by an awareness of insecurity and doubt.

Infants persist in testing and confirming their basic assumptions about their world through play behavior. Toward the end of the first year of life, they delight in the repetition of situations that feature "predictable surprises." This is seen in simple peek-a-boo games and in toys such as jack-in-the-box. Cause-and-effect relationships are discovered, and correct assumptions about the outcome of a specific action result in great pleasure. The awareness of rhythm combined with control over the onset and speed of movement can be observed in social play. The young child enjoys the combination of sound, rhythm, and movement when playing pat-a-cake. These few examples illustrate the interaction of sensory, motor, cognitive, and social development expressed as part of play development that supports a foundation of trust in oneself and one's perception of the environment.

Implications

(sensorimotor)

Disabled infants have a diminished opportunity to explore their bodies and the environment. How can a 6-month-old child visually, manually, and orally explore legs and feet when the ability to move arms, legs, and pelvis against gravity is missing? When motor control proceeds abnormally, how can initially crude interaction patterns with toys be refined and adapted in response to an object's plasticity and sound potential? Abnormal neuromuscular development can interfere with postural control and thereby with the ability to attend. Deficient control of the head is a hindrance to maintaining visual contact with interesting events in the environment. Learning about the function of various objects and about basic processes of daily life is influenced by the opportunity to observe, a prerequisite for imitative and representational play. Deficits in postural control and mobility may result in many fewer models for imitative play than are available to the unimpaired child.

Therapists can be of assistance in dealing with these deficits. During treatment, infants may need time to explore their body parts, to reach for and touch a parent's face or suitable toys, and to use the relatively normal sensorimotor state for initiating interaction with the environment. Therapy can thereby support the development of trust in the competence of one's own body and in the interpretation of the environment. In order to enhance opportunities to develop knowledge about basic events of daily life, impaired infants may need to be positioned so they can regularly observe suitable activities. Such observation augments the models for basic elements of imitative and representational play as well as making an important contribution toward the foundation of communication (13).

In summary, through assistance from specific positioning, assistance with movement, and the selection of play materials that are optimal in size, shape, weight, texture, sound effect, and visual attraction, the impaired infant can have regular opportunities to engage in play activities that contribute to learning and support early play development.

The sensorimotor period (characterized by exploratory activities and the development of basic cognitive concepts and gross motor and fine motor control) builds the foundation for two types of play activities that emerge around the end of the second year of life and continue to be of importance throughout childhood: symbolic play and constructive play.

Symbolic Play

Pretending is defined by Garvey (2) as a voluntary transformation of some aspects of reality. Time, place, people, and objects may be transformed, and absent objects and people may be represented to suit an imaginary situation. A sequential increase in the complexity of representational or symbolic play can be derived from various studies (6–8, 13–18). Action models first come from the immediate environment. A child initially performs self-related activities, such as pretending to drink from an empty cup.

This is followed by pretend play that includes a doll or a person. Dolls have an initially passive role, such as being fed; later they are assigned an active role, such as feeding themselves. Pretending eventually includes activities that children have observed in others but are not yet capable of performing, for instance driving a truck or reading a book. Initially, the pretend play period is characterized by the use of fairly realistic objects. With increasing age children depend less on the external features of play material, but project onto it their own ideas (18).

Pretending starts as solitary play and develops into situations that represent complex social interaction patterns involving several children, such as playing house or school. Besides the ability to pretend and the children's mutual agreement to respect the rules of such play, organizational skills are called on in these types of play activities. For instance, pretending to cook a meal for a family usually requires that various "family" members execute specific tasks, such as shopping, cooking, or setting the table. A sense of timing and sequencing supports the success of this type of group interaction, which has been called cooperative play (19).

Symbolic play is well established in most normally developing children by the age of 3, but only around the age of 5 is it incorporated into truly cooperative play groups. According to Garvey (2), it can be observed into middle childhood and should decrease or change into daydreaming before adolescence.

Constructive Play

Constructive play develops concurrently with symbolic play. During constructive play the child responds to and works with the physical properties of reality and the characteristics of the play materials (20). The extensive exploration of the environment that began during the sensorimotor period helps the child interpret sensory stimuli, adapt motor patterns accordingly, and make fairly reliable perceptual assumptions about a material's constructive potential. For instance, the properties of wooden blocks "communicate" that they can be used for building, and the properties of wooden beads "communicate" that they can be used for threading, for rolling if they are round, or for stacking if they have two flat surfaces.

The beginning of constructive play can be observed toward the end of a child's second year. At approximately the age of 3, children begin to have the ability to form a mental image of what they are going to construct. This internal plan guides their actions (21). As children grow older, constructive play becomes more complex in regard to the materials and the construction methods employed. Based on a study of 3- to 10-year-olds, Greenfield (22) reported an increasing complexity in strategies of construction and more precision in end products.

The clearer the message from the material, the earlier it can be used for constructive play. Materials that lack distinctive form and require shaping or transforming, such as clay or drawing supplies, or materials consisting of many different pieces that require intermediate parts (such as screws) to be connected require the dexterity, skill, and ability to visualize the end product usually found in an older child. Studies that compared play behavior between middle- and lower-class preschoolers (23, 24) and between preschool and kindergarten children indicated that constructive play was more frequent in middle-class preschoolers and that kindergartners more often engaged in it than preschoolers. Apparently, a variety of factors in addition to age can influence the frequency with which children engage in specific types of play.

Transition From Early to Middle Childhood

Both symbolic and constructive play last into middle childhood, a time span that covers several of Erikson's stages (3). The stage of "Autonomy vs. Shame and Doubt" lasts approximately from ages 18 months to 3 years. Erikson discusses shame in terms of being self-conscious of unwanted total exposure, while doubt is described in relation to the space "behind" an individual and the feelings associated with having personal autonomy threatened by outside forces.

During this period, toddlers have gained basic control of their bodies in relation to gravity, and they begin to experiment with their control over the environment by asserting themselves towards others, trying out the effect of the word "no," and by testing their independence. They challenge their physical coordination and power by running, climbing, carrying, throwing, pushing, and pulling. The beginnings of symbolic and constructive play open new avenues for control. In symbolic play, children assert autonomy over reality by transforming it or by supplementing it with imagined objects or people. Through imitation, children can place themselves in the role of adults and exercise adult perogatives, such as deciding a doll's bedtime. In constructive play, control is exerted over play material by the recognition of its inherent characteristics and by its appropriate use.

This stage is followed by one labeled "Initiative vs. Guilt," characteristic of the period from approximately 3 to 6 years of age. According to Erikson (3), "Initiative adds to autonomy the quality of undertaking, planning, and 'attacking' a task for the sake of being active and on the move" (p. 255). He suggests that "the danger of this stage is a sense of guilt over the goals contemplated and the acts initiated in one's exuberant enjoyment of new locomotor and mental power" (p. 255).

In play, mental and physical skills are used to investigate the potential of various materials to construct and create. Symbolic play allows children to venture into realms that might be frightening in real life. Both in constructive activities and in symbolic play, the child's readiness to risk and to take responsibility, cooperate in, and complete short projects can be observed. To have their products saved and their efforts acknowledged is especially important to children in this stage (25).

Initiative and risk-taking also are reflected in gross motor activities. Outdoor equipment that offers an opportunity to slide, swing, hide, climb, bounce, and jump lends itself to these purposes.

Implications for the Disabled Child

(Symbolic Play and Constructive Play)

It is important to preface specific implications drawn from these aspects of development with some general observations. The chronological age of impaired children frequently is not indicative of their developmental level. There may be significant discrepancies between the functional levels at which a particular child is able to perform. Atypical differences may exist between physical abilities, sensory integration, and perceptual, cognitive, social, and communication skills. Therapists, therefore, need to have a clear idea of the level at which a child functions in each area of development. This information increases the probability of appropriate interaction and the selection of activities that meet the child's specific interests and needs.

An awareness of symbolic and constructive play development and of Erikson's stages of growth provides a basis for incorporating some aspects of normal play development into work with disabled children. Focusing on symbolic play, a therapist may question if a child has opportunities to learn from activities that could serve as models. Does the child have the perceptual and cognitive abilities to benefit from exposure to various activities? Does the child have the physical and communication skills to engage in symbolic play? As previously pointed out, adequate attending skills are a prerequisite for learning. For example, a child with predominantly abnormal postural reactions when moved or touched may be absorbed by the experience of discomfort or fear. Such a child cannot attend to potential learning situations inherent in the activities of dressing or bathing. Specific therapeutic handling during these activities can reduce the child's fear of being overwhelmed by sensory stimuli or by uncontrollable postural responses. The child is then freed to focus attention on the sensory, perceptual, and cognitive processes essential for learning.

Significant physical impairment combined with communication deficits prevents observable symbolic play. Assistance that enables some voluntary motor control or an alternative method of communication may assist a child in experiencing symbolic play activities. This may be of great importance, since imaginative play can make valuable contributions to an impaired child's sense of autonomy.

Symbolic play can also help a child prepare for or deal with a potentially frightening experience. For example, a child who must enter a hospital can lessen an apprehension of the strangers and unfamiliar instruments that may be encountered there by playing with a stethoscope or applying a cast to a doll's leg.

Imaginative play can support a child's sense of independence and offer a chance to make decisions that are not under his or her own control in real life. A 4-year-old boy who was severely physically handicapped enjoyed pretending to drive a car in therapy sessions. He would then decide that he was going to a friend's house for dinner, which would prompt a call to his mother to let her know he'd be arriving home late. In reality, of course, none of these options were open to him, due to both his age and his handicap.

The example of this young "driver" clearly illustrates the usefulness of imaginative play with mentally alert children who have significant physical impairments. Since this type of play depends primarily on a child's understanding of life and on imagination, the manipulation of complex play material is not necessary. Intricate plot lines may develop from such play, while the objects and utensils described in the story need only be mimed or replaced by easily manipulated ones. A 5-year-old athetoid girl, for example, described making ice cream for her teddy bear's birthday party. The interest and motivation sparked by the pretended activity led to a spontaneous repetition of movement sequences that might have seemed boring to her if presented simply as exercises. In addition, perceptual, language, and cognitive concepts were reinforced in the process of this imaginative play.

Among the prerequisites of constructive play are the perceptual and cognitive abilities to interpret relevant characteristics of play materials. The pool of information gathered from earlier sensorimotor experiences and the investigation of appropriate material usually provide the foundations for constructive play. Factors that may interfere with such constructive play are a lack of exposure to the material; an inability to manipulate material due to motor deficits; an inability to derive meaningful sensorimotor information from exposure to play material; an inability to visualize how the material can be used; or insufficient organizational skills to carry out a project.

In order to incorporate constructive activities into therapy to assist children in developing constructive play skills, it is important to observe interaction patterns with play materials and to analyze the reasons for deficits. Decreased or abnormal sensorimotor experiences are often important reasons for deficient play behavior. Children, therefore, frequently need to go through some steps of sensorimotor exploration in order to pave the way for a basic understanding of a play material's constructive potential. It is important to remember, however, that a lack of physical contact with and manipulation of the environment and play material does not necessarily result in a deficient formation of concepts or a faulty understanding of a material's inherent constructive potential.

Clinical experience with some children with severe impairments has led to the assumption that there must be ways of learning that do not primarily rely on typical sensorimotor exploration, but instead appear to employ primarily visual and auditory input for relevant information. These observations are usually based on experiences with a few athetoid children. Kopp and Shaperman's (26) case report of a young boy born without limbs provides an illustration of another atypical way of learning. They indicated that the boy developed conceptual and linguistic abilities despite the absence of manipulation and suggested that his distance receptors facilitated learning. These clinical observations should caution therapists from overgeneralizing about the ill effects of absent or abnormal sensorimotor experiences.

In order to optimize children's chances for success in constructive play, their minds should be free for creative processes. Attention should not be absorbed by excessive efforts to maintain postural control or to handle material. Therefore, the child's position and the selection and presentation of materials deserves careful consideration. Children with problems in organizing their actions may be better able to engage in basic constructive activities when the chances of chaos are minimized. This can be achieved by limiting the number and intensity of stimuli to which they are exposed, such as handing blocks to a child one by one. A therapist can also abstain from any unnecessary talking, so that the child does not have to process auditory input when full attention should be focused on the constructive process.

In assessing symbolic and constructive play, it is also necessary to differentiate between appropriate repetitions and stereotypical perseveration of play behaviors. Krakow and Kopp (27) observed that the most marked difference in the quality of play behaviors between unimpaired and developmentally delayed young children was the frequency of inflexibly repetitive activities, accompanied by little social interaction with their mothers. The repetitive bathing and feeding of a doll were cited as examples of such behavior.

Strategies that Foster Control

Impaired children may experience the urge for control and autonomy, but their options to express these needs are restricted. Nonambulatory children and children who lack adequate communication skills are especially dependent on others. Play activities that include possibilities for direct control over events in the environment may support the development of a sense of autonomy in such children. Cause and effect relationships, in which children find themselves in control of an event, can be very satisfying. For instance, setting a toy car in motion by pushing it down an incline requires little physical skill but has an obvious result.

Having control over one's own movement in the environment is an important experience. Butler's (28) study demonstrated that through the use of motorized wheelchairs, children as young as 24 months were able to achieve independent mobility. She also reports positive effects on such children's social, emotional, and intellectual behavior.

A sense of control may also help in reducing the fear of unfamiliar equipment. For instance, some children accept being placed and moved on mobile equipment more easily after first touching and pushing the apparatus themselves.

The need for a sense of control, of course, does not vanish at the end of the "Autonomy vs. Shame and Doubt" stage. Play activities and other situations throughout the day should reinforce the concept that a child's actions and decisions have consistent consequences and influence events in the environment. This may prevent behaviors typical of "learned helplessness," such as a lack of motivation in problem solving (29).

The "Initiative vs. Guilt" stage emphasizes the importance of situations that allow children to express and experiment with their own ideas and action patterns. The therapy situation primarily seeks to influence a child's actions and reactions in order to decrease the limiting aspects of abnormal motor and behavioral patterns. Increasing flexible options to act on and interact with the environment is another typical goal. Through play activities, the therapist can often both modify a child's action patterns and enhance the child's self-confidence in problem-solving abilities. An obstacle course that requires motor planning and movement patterns appropriate for a child's functional level or experimenting with mixing paint colors to make hand- and footprints with the help of a therapist are examples of such activities.

Rule Games

Garvey (2) points out that the English language differentiates between *play* and *game*, whereas in German and French a single word encompasses both meanings. She describes games as a form of play activities that have become institutionalized. Precise rules that can be learned are an important characteristic. Precursors of rule games can be found in early social interactions, such as peek-a-boo games. Bruner and Sherwood (30) studied mother-infant pairs and described how both participants showed respect for each other's specific roles in such games by repeatedly adhering to specific movement and communication patterns. A different sense of rule acknowledgment is seen in constructive play, as children work within the inherent rules of the play materials.

The ability to competently participate in rule games appears around the age of 5 to 6 years (2). It requires a combination of skills including memory, organization, planning, sequencing, and the ability to focus on details without losing sight of the whole. Initially, rule games with peers tend to be cooperative (for instance, ring-around-the-roses), while later they become competitive, which means that children at times have to deal with being on the losing side.

At the same approximate time that rule games begin to be important, Erikson's (3) last preadolescent stage, "Industry vs. Inferiority," occurs. It covers the period from approximately 6 to 12 years. By now children have the physical dexterity and cognitive skills that contribute to a sense of competence and achievement. The skilled use of tools helps produce things that earn recognition. Children may spend considerable time working on individual or group projects, at school or in groups such as scouting organizations. Feelings of inadequacy and inferiority may be caused by lack of skills in the use of tools or by dissatisfaction with end products. Inadequate performance and unsatisfactory results may lead to a decrease in a child's self-esteem and a lowering of peer status.

Implications

Many rule games, such as chess, require physical and mental abilities that are complex. The combination of pleasure, social skills, and learning that these games can promote emphasizes the need for adapting them for children with disabilities who have the mental abilities to participate successfully. Magnetic chessboards, for example, can reduce the chance that pieces fall as a result of involuntary movement. Play figures can be stabilized on a pegboard. Large dice can facilitate grasp and release. Games with easy-to-comprehend rules make participation possible for some children with mental and physical deficits. Enlarged game boards can assist in reducing visual confusion and the need for fine motor control.

Appropriate adaptations also offer disabled and nondisabled people a chance to play together on equal terms. Such adaptations also provide an opportunity to demonstrate mental abilities that may far exceed motor skills. The ability to pariticipate in rule games also provides choices for future leisure activities. A popular contemporary form of rule games are computer games, and the possibilities for their adaptation to various physical and cognitive levels expand continuously and promise new options for the future (31).

Disabled children need the opportunity to experience a true sense of succcess not only in board games but in a wide range of activities throughout the preadolescent "Industry vs. Inferiority" stage. While such opportunities may be scarce, they do exist in recreational activities (32–35) such as swimming and horseback riding in addition to the previously discussed adapted constructive activities and rule games. Acquiring the skill to use a computer not only provides satisfaction in itself, but also can give a child a tool to explore and express a variety of hidden abilities.

Children at this stage of development typically judge their own performance against that of their peers. Telling a child that his or her handmade product is beautiful when it actually falls far short of expectations does not contribute to building a realistic sense of self-worth. Therapists face the challenge of identifying both play and non-play activities that help disabled children to gain a genuine sense of achievement—one that will not collapse when confronted with the standards, the competence, and the products of the "unimpaired world."

Play and Therapy, Play or Therapy?

Conclusion

In summary, therapy goals often fail to gain an impaired child's attention or cooperation because they tend to be too remote or abstract to be experienced as intrinsically motivating. Play, by contrast, offers just such an intrinsic motivation. The impaired child's deficits, however, may often interfere with play, or play itself may conflict with the process of achieving therapy goals. Play activities, then, can bridge this gap between play and therapy. A therapist familiar with both play and personality development can integrate play behavior into specific therapeutic activities, making those activities relevant and rewarding for children. Play activities, however, should neither be used primarily as a device to disguise therapy nor held as a reward until the completion of a session. When properly conceived and utilized, play activities have the power to translate the multifaceted aspects of environmental interaction into experiences that are directly meaningful to the child in the "here and now." Thus, rewarding engagement in play activities in the present can contribute to future achievements.

References

1. Chance P: *Learning Through Play*. Pediatric round table series #3. New Brunswick, NJ: Johnson & Johnson Baby Products, 1979
2. Garvey C: *Play*. London: Fontana/Open Books Publishing, 1977
3. Erikson EH: *Childhood and Society*, 2nd Edition. New York: Norton & Co, 1963
4. Kravitz H, Goldenberg D, Neyhus A: Tactual exploration by normal infants. *Dev Med Child Neurol* 20:720–726, 1978
5. Rosenblatt D: Developmental trends in infant play. In *Biology of Play*, B Tizard, D Harvey, Editors. Clinics in Developmental Medicine, No. 62. London: Heinemann, 1977
6. Belsky J, Most RK: From exploration to play: A cross-sectional study of infant free play behavior. *Developmental Psychology* 17:630–639, 1981.
7. Largo RH, Howard JA: Developmental progression in play behaviors of children between nine and thirty months. I. Spontaneous play and initiation. *Dev Med Child Neurol* 21:299–310, 1979
8. McCune-Nicolich L: Beyond sensorimotor intelligence: Assessment of symbolic maturity through analysis of pretend play. *Merrill-Palmer Quarterly* 23:89–99, 1977
9. Lezine, I: The transition from sensory-motor to earliest symbolic function in early development. *Early Development*, Research Publication ARNMD, 51:221–232, 1973
10. McCall R: Exploratory manipulation and play in the human infant. *Monogr Soc Res Child Dev* 39, pp. 21–25, 1974
11. Fenson L, Kagan J, Kearsley RB, Zelazo PR: The developmental progression of manipulative play in the first two years. *Child Dev* 47:232–236, 1976
12. Bruner JS: Organization of early skilled action. *Child Dev* 44:1–11, 1973
13. McCune-Nicolich L: Toward symbolic functioning: Structure of early pretend games and potential parallels with language. *Child Dev* 52:785–797, 1981

14. Lowe M: Trends in the development of representational play in infants from one to three years—An observational study. *Child Psychology and Psychiatry* 16:33–47, 1975
15. Fenson L, Ramsey DS: Decentration and integration of child's play in the second year. *Child Dev* 51:171–178, 1980
16. Fein G: A transitional analysis of pretending. *Developmental Psychology* 11:291–296, 1975
17. Fein, GG: Pretend play in childhood: An integrative review. *Child Dev* 52:1095–1118, 1981
18. Elder J, Pederson D: Preschool children's use of objects in symbolic play. *Child Dev.* 49:500–504, 1978
19. Parten MB: Social play among preschool children. In *Child's Play*, RE Herron, B Sutton-Smith, Editors. New York: John Wiley & Sons, 1971
20. Rast M: The use of play activities in therapy. *Developmental Disabilities Special Interest Section Newsletter* 7:1, 4, 1984
21. Moor P: *Die Bedeutung des Spieles in der Erziehung*. Bern: Huber, 1972
22. Greenfield PM: Building a tree structure: The development of hierarchical complexity and interrupted strategies in children's construction activity. *Developmental Psychology* 13:299–313, 1977
23. Rubin KH, Maioni TL, Horning M: Free play behaviors in middle and lower-class preschoolers: Parten & Piaget revisited. *Child Dev* 47:414–419, 1976
24. Rubin KH, Watson KS, Jambor TW: Free-play behavior in preschool and kindergarten children. *Child Dev* 49:534–536, 1978
25. Takata N: Play as a prescription. In *Play as Exploratory Learning*, M Reilly, Editor. Beverly Hills: Sage Publications, 1974
26. Kopp CB, Shaperman J: Cognitive development in the absence of object manipulation during infancy. *Developmental Psychology* 9:430, 1973
27. Krakow JB, Kopp CB: The effects of developmental delay on sustained attention in young children. *Child Dev* 54:1143–1155, 1983
28. Butler C, Okamoto GA, McKay TM: Powered mobility for very young disabled children. *Dev Med Child Neurol* 25:472–474, 1983
29. Alloy LB, Seligman MEP: On the cognitive component of learned helplessness and depression. *Psychology of Learning and Motivation* 13:219–276, 1979
30. Bruner JS, Sherwood V: Peekaboo and the learning of rule structures. In *Play, Its Role in Development and Evolution*, JS Bruner, A Jolly, K Sylva, Editors. New York: Basic Books, 1976
31. Kee DW: Computer Play. In *Play Interactions: The Role of Toys and Parental Involvement in Children's Development*, Caldwell Brown C, Gottfried AW (Editors) Pediatric round table series #11, New Brunswick, NJ: Johnson & Johnson Baby Products, 1985 pp. 53–60
32. Martin K: Therapeutic pool activities for young children in a community facility. *Physical and Occupational Therapy in Pediatrics* 3:59–74, 1983
33. Harris SR: Neurodevelopmental treatment approach for teaching swimming to cerebral palsied children *Phys Ther.* 58:938–979, 1978
34. Harris SR, Thompson M: Water as a learning environment for facilitating gross motor skills in deaf-blind children. *Physical and Occupational Therapy in Pediatrics* 3:75–82, 1983
35. Klein MM: The therapeutics of recreation. *Physical and Occupational Therapy in Pediatrics* 4:9–11, 1984

4. Who Do You Want To Be Today?

The Use of Costumes as Dressing Training in Occupational Therapy

Jean Douglas Clarkson

Jean Douglas Clarkson, OTR, is a member of the staff at Durant-Tuuri-Mott School in Flint, Michigan, where she works primarily with preschool physically handicapped children. She has received funding for programs in dressing, home programs, positioning, movement, and adapted toys. She was formerly the head of Occupational Therapy at Winchester Hospital, Flint, Michigan; a homebound occupational therapist at the Michigan Society for Crippled Children and Adults; and a staff therapist at Kalamazoo (Michigan) State Hospital. She received her BS in occupational therapy from Western Michigan University and has done graduate work at Eastern Michigan University and Wayne State University.

Who Do You Want To Be Today?

Play, according to Hendrick (1), offers children the opportunity to achieve mastery of their environment. In turn, pretended and actual mastery foster the growth of ego strength in young children. Creative play is expressed in two ways: through the unusual use of familiar materials and equipment, and through role playing and imaginative play (1). When a child first tries on father's hat, he or she begins to role play, a process of recreating the world through his or her own imagination. Children with physical handicaps are limited in this, as they are in other forms of play. They may not be able to move well enough to explore their environment. If they can get into closets, they may not have the coordination to pull on father's hat or mother's shoes. For them, their lack of skill may make dressing a chore rather than a challenge.

The occupational therapist saw these limitations in the 3-, 4-, and 5-year-olds entering the preschool classroom for Physically or Otherwise Health Impaired (POHI) at the Durant-Tuuri-Mott School in Flint, Michigan. Most of the children were diagnosed having cerebral palsy. Many could not remove their coats or handle their clothes when toileting. Some could select and play with toys independently during free play, while others were limited in this activity. The teacher presented the children with regular dress-up clothes, but they did not attempt to try them on or participate in dramatic play. Parent expectations were low. In occupational therapy, the children first used their own clothing to practice dressing skills. Because the task of dressing was difficult for them, they often resisted this activity and spent most of the therapy time in getting their clothes off, which meant we had to dress them hurriedly at the end of a session. Montessori boards and practice shoes helped develop skills but did not motivate the children. It also became apparent that dressing training needed to be made relevant to the children's own lives. During an evaluation, for example, one occupational therapist helped a little boy remove his clothing. When he finished, and expecting him to begin to dress, she asked, "Now what do we do?" "Go to bed!" he replied. Struck with his logic, the therapist began to look for more meaningful ways to teach dressing skills.

Use of Costumes in Dressing Training

Costumes had been previously used for dressing training with the children, and they seemed to enjoy dressing up and role playing. Two garments were already favorites: a button-up felt cowboy vest and a Ronald McDonald shirt. However, the fabrics used in their construction proved unsatisfactory. The felt stretched at the buttonholes and was not washable, and the shirt's woven fabric was hard to pull over clothing.

One day, Jeremy, a boy with congenital deformities, came to Swim Day in a blue stretch terry cloth outfit. He quickly learned to pull off the shirt and pants by himself, and after a few sessions, he learned to pull them on again. The therapist realized that stretch terry cloth costumes would be helpful for dressing train-

Jean Douglas Clarkson

ing. With the soft stretch fabric, the children could easily pull on the costumes over their clothing, eliminating the need to undress. The costumes could also be washed when soiled. Using them, the children could learn dressing skills in a simple and fun way.

The Flint Board of Education offered minigrants for innovative teaching ideas, and the therapist submitted a request for $75.00 to purchase fabric and patterns and provide inservice training on dressing techniques for parents. With the grant, she purchased stretch terry cloth in bright colors and two commercial patterns in sizes 4 to 6.

The classroom teacher and the swimming instructor helped the therapist to compile a booklet of dressing tips, which was printed with minigrant funds and distributed to parents at an afternoon inservice training session. At the session, a sewing teacher demonstrated stretch fabric sewing techniques, and parents viewed a display of clothing with simple fasteners from a local store.

Volunteers helped the therapist sew costumes for superheroes and imaginary characters. These were hung on a low rack in a corner of the occupational therapy room, near a mirror and a child-size table and chairs. Hats and masks hung invitingly from a screen. Volunteers and occupational therapy students in clinical training at the center often construct new costumes to add to the collection. Other outfits are donated after Halloween each year. A dance instructor gave a box of stretchy costumes with bright ruffled net tutus and fancy hats.

Costumed dramatic play, as pointed out by Ames and Ilg (2), is age-appropriate for the preschool child. Children at this age

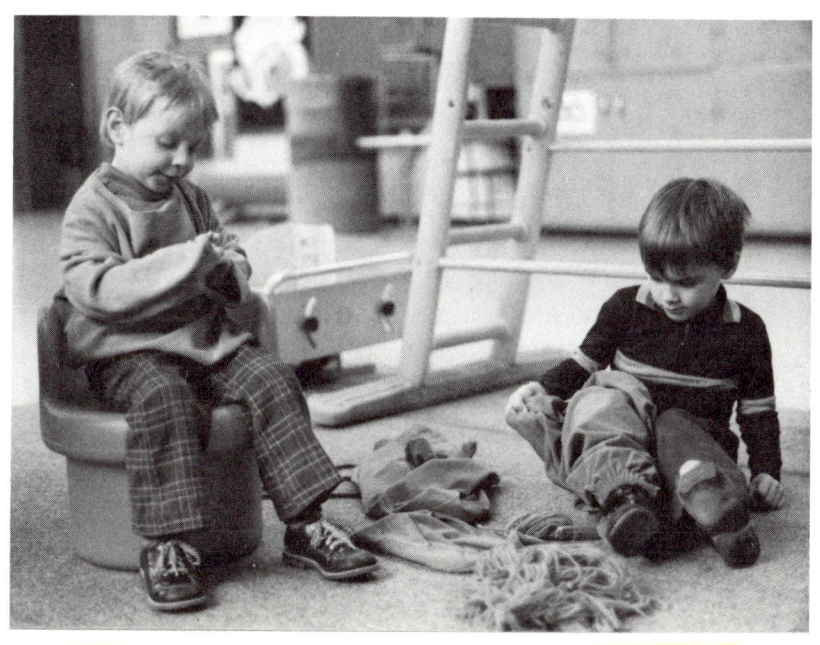

Costumes that are easy to put on can encourage preschoolers in developing dressing skills.

Who Do You Want To Be Today?

take a special delight in role playing, in acting out behaviors seen in the adult: feeding a child, talking on the phone, or even sweeping the floor (2).

These behaviors do not happen as spontaneously with physically handicapped children, however. They often develop a "learned helplessness" and appear to require more assistance in role play. Thus, the therapist leads the child to the rack and often guides the selection of a costume appropriate for the child's skills.

Individual Evaluation

Before dressing training begins, the occupational therapist evaluates the child's level of function by marking a chart (see Table 1) as the child undresses and dresses. Color coding indicates the child's level of skill. Green denotes skills performed independently; yellow indicates areas where help is needed; and red points out skills that cannot yet be performed. Those skills marked in yellow are target areas for dressing training. The chart is detailed to pinpoint present levels of function and indicate progress on each reevaluation. In six months, a child may still be unable to put on a shirt independently, but the chart may show progress from "grasp and pull" to "pull over head" and "on one arm."

Murphy and associates (3) point out that although physically handicapped children may not learn spontaneously as normal children, they need to be taught according to the normal progression. Normal children do not begin dressing until about 18 months of age when they can sit unsupported in a chair and have mastered fine coordinated movements (3). The following progression of skills in the normal child has been outlined by Gesell (4):

- 18 months: Begins putting on hat, socks, mittens.
- 2 years: Removes shoes, socks, and pants; likes to undress.
- 2½ years: Takes off all clothes and can put on socks, shirt, and coat, although not always accurately.
- 3 years: Undresses rapidly and well, including buttons; able to dress except for heavy outer clothing; cannot tell front from back.
- 4 years: Dresses and undresses with little assistance; can tell front from back.

Training Examples

Children tend to approach dressing with similar patterns. In attempting to pull off a sock, the beginner usually grasps the toe and pulls. When removing a pullover shirt, the child usually tugs at the wrist or pulls the shirt over the head toward the back of the neck. The child often grasps pants from the front with no awareness of his or her back.

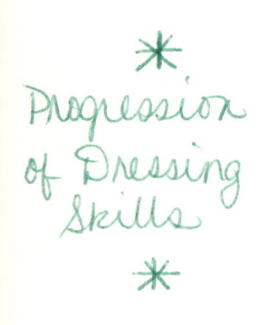

Therapists need to teach more useful methods, such as grasping the sock cuff with the thumb and fingers of both hands and pulling over the heel, grasping a shirt under the arm and pulling out the elbow, pulling a shirt over the back of the head before pulling it over the face, and grasping pants with both hands, pulling from sides and back. Skill with pants develops as the child becomes toilet trained; skill with shirts lags behind.

Costumes help teach these dressing skills. The simplest outfits are sleeveless and can be pulled over the head and off easily. A child who masters this can try on the stretch outfits with sleeves, pant legs, and elastic waistbands. The child who is ready to learn how to fasten buttons and ties can learn these skills with more complex costumes. (See Table 2 for the costumes used in the program and specific skill levels.)

The costume rack holds a variety of garments for various skill levels. The most successful costumes are those that the children readily recognize, such as superheroes and Strawberry Shortcake. These are made from stretch materials in sizes slightly larger than the child's own clothing. Children get lost inside a shirt that is too large and in which they cannot find the armhole. Clothing that is too small is equally difficult. Sizes 4 to 6 in commercial patterns fit most of the children learning to dress in the program.

Children can use a costume in a variety of ways. Troy, a 4-year-old with limited function due to cerebral palsy, can pull an appliquéd astronaut bib over his face. Then he pretends to be an astronaut as he spoon-feeds himself, splashes paint on paper at the easel, or propels himself in the net swing. The costume supplies a cover-up and encourages imaginative play.

Amber, a 4-year-old with cerebral palsy, was ambulatory but sluggish in dressing. She enjoyed pulling on the two-piece Holly Hobby dress and adding a fox mask under her bonnet before parading down the hall to show off. When she gained more skill through putting on costumes, she began to do more of her own dressing at home and after swimming.

Christina, a 6-year-old with Huntington's chorea, became so withdrawn that she seldom spoke. The therapist helped her dress in a princess costume and handed her a star-tipped wand. Christina waved her wand, granting wishes to each staff member she met. She became so animated in her role as a fairy godmother that she did not want to take off her costume at the end of the therapy session.

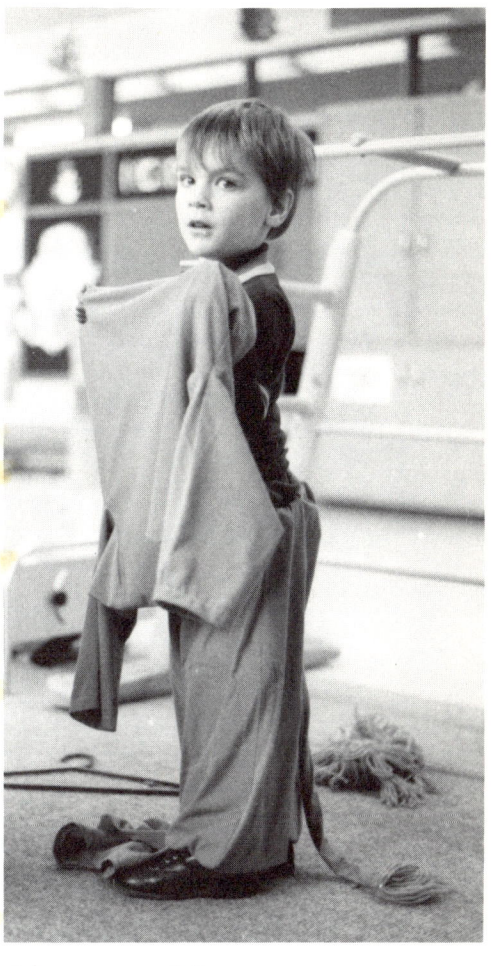

Sometimes, the therapist has to guide children away from the costumes. Brian, a 6-year-old with cerebral palsy, made a beeline for the Superman costume at every session. The costume encouraged him to use his involved right hand as he pulled himself on the scooter board or propelled himself in the swing, but he also needed other activities to develop his fine motor skills. The dress-up activity was reserved to reward him at the end of the session when he had completed his assigned fine motor tasks.

When a child returns to show off for the teacher, the costumes find their way into classrooms. At Halloween, the POHI children borrow outfits for their parties. During Circus Week, the POHI preschoolers held a parade through the school, supplementing costumes the teacher brought with the therapists' clown suits, lion outfit, and spangled dance costumes. The therapist also takes costumes into the classroom to teach dressing and social interaction through modified relay races.

Supplementary Aids

In addition to the costumes, the therapist uses various aids to teach skill with fasteners, such as a vest with a large zipper, Dressy Bessy and Dapper Dan dolls, and snap blocks. Fisher Price Button-Ups promote simple in-and-out buttoning skills and can be used to teach pattern matching. Children often remove their shoes and socks for sensory integration activities such as the climber and trampoline, and they practice putting them on afterward. For tying, we use a large cord that the child learns to tie around his or her waist, a lacing shoe, and a therapist-made booklet, entitled *Tie the Bunny's Ears*. Crafts such as macramé and yarn pom-pom animals offer additional knot-tying practice. Hoops are slipped over head, hands, and feet.

Dan Stocks, OTR, added another dimension to our dressing program during his internship when he constructed Rita, a life-size fabric doll who can wear costumes. Rita is a guest at every tea party, and the children change her outfits regularly. She can often be found seated at the table, in the swing, or at the therapist's desk. Rita gives the children an opportunity to solve problems as they try to stuff her arms into shirt sleeves or her legs into pants. She is especially useful with children who are reluctant to dress themselves.

Preschool POHI teacher Jane Somers was inspired by costume kits at a local nursery school that could be used in occupational therapy and in the classroom. Therapists and teachers can develop collections around a number of themes:

Doctor Box—white shirts, nurses' caps, bandages, stethoscope.

Beauty Shop—wigs, wig stands, curlers, combs, old hair dryers, capes.

Grocery Store—cash register, cans, aprons, market basket, purses.

Pizza Parlor—aprons, chef's hat, order pad, felt "pizzas" to assemble.

King and Queen—crowns, jewelry, robes.

Imaginative materials encourage children to put together their own outfits. These could include fur scarves, old hats and caps, gloves, high-heeled shoes, boots, capes, and fabric strips for sashes or scarves. Hendrick (1) states that costumes can enhance play, but unstructured material that can be used in many ways is even more desirable, since it helps children to be inventive and imaginative. A scarf, for example, can become a hat, an apron, a blanket, or even a child's wished-for long hair.

Conclusion

Costumes motivate children effectively at our center to attempt dressing tasks they were formerly reluctant to perform, while assisting them in learning skills with clothing and fasteners. This paper addresses only the use of costumes with preschool physically handicapped children with normal intelligence. Further research needs to be done with other populations, such as retarded children, to determine if other children's needs could be met by using costumes to stimulate imaginative play and teach dressing skills.

Children need independence. Hendrick (1) reminds us that becoming increasingly independent is a basic goal for early childhood years and that dressing is part of the independence for which children, their parents, and their teachers strive. Occupational therapists can foster that independence by raising both the child's expertise and the parents' expectations.

References

1. Hendrick J: *The Whole Child, New Trends in Early Education*, 2nd edition. St Louis: Mosby, 1980
2. Ames L, Ilg F: *Your Two Year Old*. Gesell Institute of Child Development. New York: Dell 1980
3. Murphy M, Miller A, Stewart M, Jantzen A: Dressing techniques for the cerebral palsied child. *Am J Occup Ther* 7:8–10, 37–38, 1954
4. Gesell A, Ilg F: *The Child From Five to Ten*. New York: Harper and Brothers, 1946

Who Do You Want To Be Today?

Table 1 Dressing Skills Chart	UNDRESSING	DATE								
	Pullover shirt:									
	Grasp and pull									
	Pull off face									
	off head									
	off hands									
	off 1 arm									
	Tee shirt off									
	Top shirt off									
	Button-front shirt:									
	Grasp and pull									
	Off 1 arm									
	Off both arms									
	Pants:									
	Grasp and pull									
	Pull off hip									
	Pull to knee									
	to ankle									
	Underpants off									
	Loose pants off									
	Regular pants off									
	Socks:									
	Pull off toe									
	off heel									
	Socks off									
	Shoes:									
	Untie									
	Pull off toes									
	Off if loosened									
	Shoes off									
	Fasteners:									
	Open Velcro									
	Unzip									
	Unbutton—large									
	—small									
	Unsnap									
	Unbuckle									

Jean Douglas Clarkson

DRESSING	DATE									
Pullover shirt:										
Grasp and pull										
Pull on face										
on head										
on hands										
on 1 arm										
Tee shirt on										
Top shirt on										
Button-front shirt:										
Grasp and pull										
1 arm in										
Both arms in										
Pants:										
Grasp and pull										
Pull knee–hip										
knee–waist										
ankle–waist										
Underpants on										
Loose pants on										
Regular pants on										
Socks:										
Pull up fr. ankle										
over heel										
over toes										
Both socks on										
Shoes:										
Put toes in										
heels in										
On if loosened										
Shoes on										
Fasteners:										
Close Velcro										
Zip—pull zipper										
—separating										
Buttons—large										
—small										
Snaps										
Buckles										

Color Code:
Green: Independent
Yellow: Needs assistance
Red: Cannot perform

Focus therapy on Yellow (needs assistance)

Table 2
Using Costumes to Teach Specific Skills

Costume	Construction Details	Skills
Astronaut Bib	Bath towel with ribbing sewn around opening for head, appliqués of stars and stripes	Pull on, off head
Smurf	Blue turtleneck dickey with Smurf appliqué	Pull on, off head
	White stocking cap	Pull hat on, off
Strawberry Shortcake	Red turtleneck dickey	Pull on, off head
	Pink hat with polka dot brim, fringe	Pull hat on, off
	Short red skirt with elasticized waistband	Skirt on, off
	Red vest with strawberry appliqué, large button closure	Arms in armholes Buttoning
Clown	Ring of fabric, gathered on elastic	Pull on, off head
	Clown hat, yarn wig	Pull hat on, off
	One piece clown suit, open front with tie closure	Pull on one-piece garment; tying bow
Superman, Batman	Stretch terry cloth shirts with appliqués	Shirt on, off
	Stretch terry cloth pants with elasticized waistbands	Pants on, off
	Capes with ties	Tying bow
Holly Hobby	Printed double-knit pullover top with lace trimming	Shirt on, off
	Long skirt with elasticized waistband	Skirt on, off
	Bonnet with ties	Hat on, off Tying bow
Princess	Long pullover Quiana dress, elasticized neck and waist, beaded trim, long sleeves	Dress on, off
	Silver cardboard crown, wand	Hat on, off
Cowboy	Vest with large armholes	Arms in armholes
	Vest buttons at shoulder with small buttons, larger buttons for front closure, button-on star	Use of buttons

Jean Douglas Clarkson

	Cut-off khaki pants that fasten with snap, zipper, belt	Pants on, off Use of fasteners
	Optional snap-front shirt	Arms in sleeves Use of fasteners
Dance	Skirt-length net ruffle gathered on elasticized waist	Legs in skirts
	Stretch fabric dance costumes with sequin trim	Legs in openings, arms in armholes
Jewelry	Beads strung on elastic thread Plastic necklace with charms	Pull on, off head
	Plastic bangle bracelets	Pull on, off hands

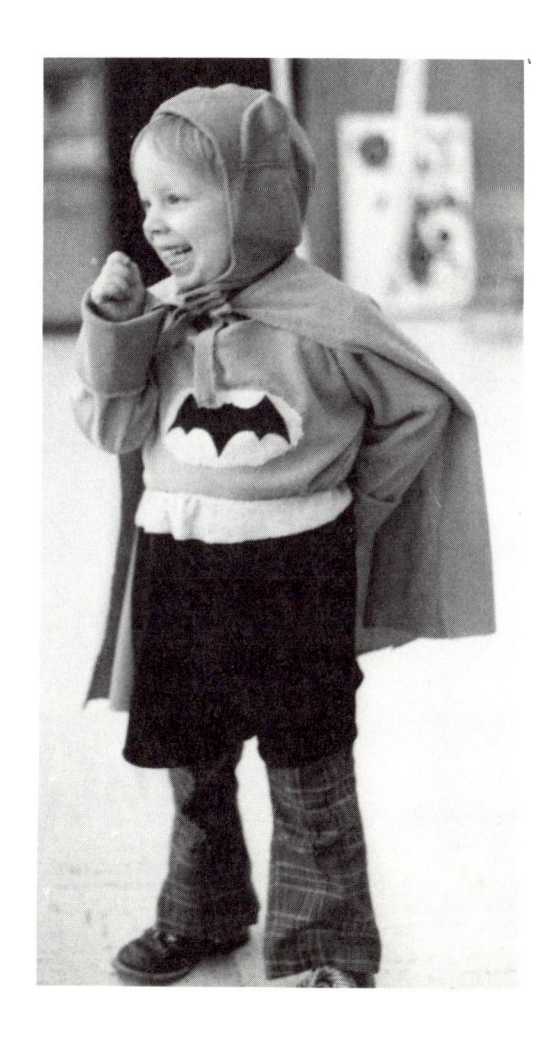

53

5.
Infant Play: A Reflection of Cognitive and Motor Development

Diane D'Eugenio

Diane D'Eugenio, MA, OTR, is a graduate of the University of New Hampshire and the University of Michigan. While in Michigan, she worked on a federally funded project designed to develop and disseminate a model for early intervention services. A clinical assistance professor in the Department of Pediatrics at the State University of New York's Upstate Medical Center in Syracuse, she works with premature infants on a neonatal intensive care unit, in follow-up, and as part of the staff of an interdisciplinary center for the assessment of infants and children.

Infant Play: A Reflection of Cognitive and Motor Development

"Pulls string to get a ring." "Shakes a rattle." "Stacks blocks." "Completes a pegboard."

These items on a developmental checklist are familiar to occupational therapists who evaluate and treat infants. They represent milestones for which objectives are created, assessments are made, and actions are integrated into treatment activities. But what do these descriptions actually represent, and why are these activities characteristic of all children at a certain developmental level?

Training in neuromotor development enables occupational therapists to answer questions about the specific motor skills involved in shaking a rattle or stacking a set of blocks. An understanding of a child's emotional needs, relationship with parents, individual temperament, and environmental influences fosters a sensitivity to the effects that psychosocial factors have on play.

But play is also a child's expression of cognitive development. It serves as a means of exploring the environment and understanding the world. Play is a window through which we can see the dynamic formation of a child's cognitive concepts and the elaboration and refinement of those concepts over time. By integrating an understanding of this cognitive dimension of play with its neuromotor and psychosocial elements, occupational therapists can approach evaluation and treatment planning with a more comprehensive, more complete base of information from which to write appropriate treatment objectives.

This chapter focuses on the cognitive dimension of play through a review of Jean Piaget's theory of the sensorimotor period of cognitive development. Accompanying tables present the relationship between the underlying cognitive and motor components of a number of familiar play items. Methods by which this information can be applied in developmental assessments and treatment plans for infants who are developmentally disabled are presented.

Piaget's Sensorimotor Period of Cognitive Development

The sensorimotor period is the first of four separate cognitive periods identified by Piaget. Its six stages describe a child's development from simple biological reflexes to the emergence of representational thought.

It should be remembered that this chapter covers only the highlights of this component of Piaget's theory of intellectual development. Specific aspects of the sensorimotor period are examined as they relate to the development of certain themes within a young child's play. These include the development of imitation skills, knowledge of object constancy, spatial relationships, and causality.

The age ranges indicated for each of the six stages are simply guidelines, chronological boundaries that vary from child to child. However, the order of the stages and the sequence in which a child passes through them remain constant (1).

Stage 1: Reflexive (Birth–1 month)

A newborn's movements are dominated by reflexes. Within a short time, some of these primary reflexes identified by Piaget—sucking, grasp, and eye movements—undergo small changes as a result of interaction with the environment. For example, after initially awkward feeding attempts, an infant's sucking reflex accommodates (adapts) to the type of nipple on which feeding is performed, which allows for greater efficiency (2). It is through the interaction of these reflex behaviors with the environment that initial changes and expansions of internal mental structures, or schemas, occur and new behaviors form (3).

Stage 2: Primary Circular Reaction (1–4 months)

At this stage, infants repeat simple behaviors in order to sustain sensory feedback. These behaviors originate from reflex motivations that are expanded and changed as a result of contact with the environment. Repeated movements evolve into habits, which become new internal mental structures or schemas. Continued environmental reaction causes new experiences to be assimilated into existing schemas, with schemas changed to accommodate the new information.

Such primary circular reactions include repeated stretching, opening and closing of the hand to feel a surface, and fingering of the hands at midline—all behaviors that generate and sustain sensory feedback.

Behavioral awareness in infants is limited to this sensory level. An infant is unaware, for example, that repeated kicking, performed solely for tactile and kinesthetic feedback, may also cause a crib mobile to move. No connections are yet made between physical action and environmental reaction.

Table 1
Examples of Cognitive and Motor Components of Developmental Items for Stage 1

Item	Underlying Cognitive Component	Underlying Motor Component
Responds to different light intensities (E)	Reflexive response	Reflexive response
Focuses momentarily on face or soft light (E)	Reflex adaptation	Reflex response to light source
Sucks well from bottle or breast (E)	Reflex adaptation	Coordination of sucking, swallowing, and breathing
Momentary regard of red ring (B)	Reflexive adaptation	Beginning control of extraocular muscles

E: Item from the Early Intervention Developmental Profile
B: Item from the Bayley Scales of Infant Development

Table 2
Examples of Cognitive and Motor Components of Developmental Items for Stage 2

Item	Underlying Cognitive Component	Underlying Motor Component
Moves head to track moving object (E)	Coordination of Schemas	Beginning head control
Turns head to sound of bell (B)	Coordination of Schemas	Beginning head control
Simple play with rattle (B)	Coordination of Schemas and Primary Circular Reaction	Grasp reflex → beginning of voluntary grasp
Fingers own hands in play at midline (E)	Primary Circular Reaction	Integration of ATNR and TLR → development of a symmetrical posture
Exploitive string play (B)	Primary Circular Reaction	Development of voluntary hand opening and closing
Supine: kicks feet alternately (E)	Primary Circular Reaction	Crossed extension reflex → symmetrical kicking → alternate kicking

E: Item from the Early Intervention Developmental Profile
B: Item from the Bayley Scales of Infant Development

The coordination or combination of schemas begins at this stage of cognitive development. The major combinations that occur are vision and hearing, suck prehension, and visual prehension (2), more commonly referred to as sound localization, hand-to-mouth behavior, and visually directed reaching.

Imitation skills also emerge at this developmental stage. An infant may now be capable of echoing a repeated sound, such as cooing, but the extent of this ability is limited by a relatively small vocal and motor repertoire.

Stage 3: Secondary Circular Reaction (4–8 months)

Unlike the previous stage in which movement is sustained solely for sensory feedback, infants are now oriented to the effects that their behavior produces on the environment. Now, for example, a baby may repeatedly kick not only for sensory feedback, but also to set a crib mobile in motion.

It is important to note that the discovery of this cause-and-effect behavior is an almost accidental one. An infant does not initially know the effect that a motor behavior will have on the environment. Rather, such relationships are established after the fact.

The progression of play with a ring and string, a toy used on developmental tests, offers a good example of this process of discovery. During the developmental stage of primary circular reaction, a baby presented with the toy will finger the string (sensory feedback) but make no connection that such manipulation will bring the ring closer. A baby in the stage of secondary circular reaction also initially plays with the string, but realizes that the ring is moving as well. The string is then pulled specifically to reach the ring.

With this new attention to causality, an entire set of play behaviors develops and dominates this stage of development. An infant no longer just mouths toys but bangs, shakes, and pats them—all actions that cause an effect in the environment and on the toy. Now infants are interested in playing with rattles, squeak toys, bells, and any other toy that can make a sound. Infants clearly signal an awareness of a cause-and-effect relationship when playing with a sound-producing toy, for once they realize that a sound stems directly from their manipulation or movement, such actions are intensified to sustain and intensify the resulting sound.

Another cognitive skill begins to emerge in this stage. It is the knowledge of object constancy or object permanence, the

Table 3
Examples of Cognitive and Motor Components of Developmental Items for Stage 3

Item	Underlying Cognitive Component	Underlying Motor Component
Bangs in play (B)	Secondary Circular Reaction	Sustained grasp and voluntary shoulder movements
Looks to the floor when something falls (E)	Beginning object constancy	Head and trunk control in upright position → independent sitting
Interest in sound production (B)	Secondary Circular Reaction	Sustained grasp and voluntary shoulder movements
Recovers rattle, in crib (B)	Beginning object constancy	Symmetrical posture in supine and hands to midline
Pulls string: secures ring (B)	Establishment of goal—post facto	Raking grasp
Imitates hand movements already in repertoire (E)	Imitation of familiar movements	Voluntary arm control

E: Item from the Early Intervention Developmental Profile
B: Item from the Bayley Scales of Infant Development

Infant Play: A Reflection of Cognitive and Motor Development

Stage 3: understanding that a person or object still exists even though it cannot be seen. In the previous stage of cognitive development, once an object was out of an infant's sight it was gone. A baby would track a spoon moved across a table, but would not look for it once it fell to the floor. A baby in the stage of secondary circular reaction will, however, look to the floor because the sound of a dropped spoon provides a clue to its location. Likewise, a baby will now retrieve a partially covered toy or pick up a rattle dropped nearby. However, no search will be made for a toy that is completely covered and gone from view. Hide a toy under a cup, for example, and the baby at this stage is more interested in the cup than in searching for the toy; the toy may be discovered inadvertently after the cup is manipulated and lifted.

At this stage, an infant's ability to imitate movements and sounds is still limited to those that can already be made. Since the number of schemas has greatly increased during this period, the number of familiar behaviors that can be imitated is much greater than in the previous stage (4).

Stage 4: Coordination of Secondary Schemas (8–12 months)

A new attention to exploring the detailed parts of toys characterizes play at this developmental stage. Whereas all toys were previously approached as if they possessed no unique physical characteristics, now a baby investigates each distinctive feature and is fascinated by detail and novelty.

This orientation to detail is reflected in a variety of ways. It is most simply manifested in a baby's visual investigation of objects or people. Picture books now command attention and a stranger may be met with a cold stare. A new toy may be slowly turned so that all of its surfaces can be investigated. More sophisticated responses depend on fine motor development. If a hand is mature enough to allow the index finger to be pointed, then the baby may poke at the details of a toy. The ability to use a fine grasp such as an inferior pincer or neat pincer grasp affords further skills for the investigation of small objects.

It is in this stage that the first separation of means from ends is seen. In the previous stage, goals were established after the fact. Now goals can be identified and followed by the combination of several schemas to achieve that goal or solve a problem. For example, now a baby presented with the ring and string immediately pulls the string to get the ring. Or if a desired toy is in view, a baby will put together several behaviors in order to get it—crawling in its direction, maneuvering around a chair in the way, and then reaching for and grasping the toy.

The concept of object constancy continues to develop. A baby who sees a toy being completely covered (what Piaget terms a single visible displacement) can retrieve it; no other visual or auditory clues to its location are now needed.

Babies now attempt to imitate new movements, even those that cannot yet be performed. While such attempts are inexact,

Table 4
Examples of Cognitive and Motor Components of Developmental Items for Stage 4

Item	Underlying Cognitive Component	Underlying Motor Component
Fingers holes in pegboard (B)	Orientation to detail	Isolation of index finger
Uncovers toy (B) Picks up cup: secures cube (B) Unwraps cube (B)	Object constancy for single visible displacements	Voluntary reach and grasp and head and trunk control in an upright position
Finger feeds small pieces of food (E)	Orientation to detail	Raking or pincer grasp
Shows knowledge of toy hidden behind a screen (E)	Object constancy, means-end, and coordination of schemas	Voluntary reach and grasp Head and trunk control → sitting Form of mobility → crawling
Stirs spoon in imitation (B) Attempts to imitate scribble (B)	Imperfect imitation of new movements	Shoulder and hand control
Puts cube in cup on command (E)	Imperfect imitation of new movements	Lack of full voluntary release → voluntary release

E: Item from the Early Intervention Developmental Profile
B: Item from the Bayley Scales of Infant Development

they may nevertheless derive great delight from them. Scribble on a piece of paper, for example, and a baby may bang a crayon in imitation of the action, absolutely pleased with the performance. This represents a major change in the learning process, because now learning can be done by imitation (2). Other changes blossom through this skill. A baby may imitate adult movements, attempt to say words, or even echo the rhythm of conversation through the use of jargon speech.

Play during this stage is dominated by experimentation. While still coordinating existing schemas, children now form new ones and solve problems through experimentation and by exploring the individual potential of an object. Although drawn by novelty and detail, a child's play in the previous stage of development did not differentiate between objects. Experimentation now focuses on forming a new schema that is appropriate to the unique properties of an object (2).

Stage 5: Tertiary Circular Response (12–18 months)

Infant Play: A Reflection of Cognitive and Motor Development

Stage 5: Spatial relationships are the most obvious area of experimentation. A child will spend endless hours filling and emptying containers, placing one object inside another, and stacking toys. All represent actions designed to explore the properties of objects and to develop new schemas that act on them.

The concept of causality develops when a child realizes that direct action on an object is not necessary to cause an effect, but that other objects or forces can precipitate an action. When presented with a raisin in a vial, a child in the previous developmental stage would try to get it out by direct action—poking, shaking, or swallowing. Now the child simply inverts the vial to release the pellet through gravity.

The concept and use of tools also emerges during this period: a child finds that a stick can help retrieve an out-of-reach toy, and the finger feeder develops into a spoon feeder.

Table 5
Examples of Cognitive and Motor Components of Developmental Items for Stage 5

Item	Underlying Cognitive Component	Underlying Motor Component
Blueboard: places 1 round block (B)	Experimentation and spatiality of objects	Controlled grasp and release
Places 1 peg repeatedly (B) Builds tower of 2 cubes (B) Closes round box (B)	Exploration of spatial relationships of objects	Refined grasp—radial grasp Voluntary release
Attains toy with stick (B)	Imitation and/or use of tool	Controlled arm movements
Retrieves raisin by inverting vial (E) Feeds self with spoon (E) Uses gestures to make wants known (B)	Use of tool	Controlled arm movements
Dangles ring by string (B) Imitates crayon stroke (B)	Imitation	Controlled arm movements and maturing grasp on tool
Repeatedly finds toy when hidden under one of several covers (E)	Object constancy for multiple visible displacements	Controlled arm movements

E: Item from the Early Intervention Developmental Profile
B: Item from the Bayley Scales of Infant Development

An interest in experimentation brings imitation skills to new levels; children also realize that their attempts at imitation are imperfect and modify them to more closely approximate the model.

The concept of object constancy also expands at this stage; a child can now locate an object after watching it placed under one of several covers.

Stage 6: Inventions of New Schemas Through Mental Combinations (18–24 months)

Thus far, each cognitive stage has been dominated by the use of motor behaviors to solve problems. This stage marks the beginning of the use of representational thought and insight learning. Mental processes now precede action. If a shelved toy is out of reach, a child will review possible problem-solving actions and perform only that one selected to help obtain the toy, such as using a chair to more easily reach the shelf. Representational thought is reflected in the ability to use words to communicate wants and to identify objects represented by black-and-white line drawings.

Cognitive abilities expand on a variety of levels. No longer does a child need to see where an object is hidden in order to find it; an image of the object can be retained as it is moved and covered. Imitative skills are immediate and precise; the child can also hold an action in memory and imitate it at a later time. Children at this stage of sensorimotor development also seek to find the cause of things. Though delighting in a wind-up toy, a child will attempt to discover the source of its motion once it has stopped.

Table 6
Examples of Cognitive and Motor Components of Developmental Items for Stage 6

Item	Underlying Cognitive Component	Underlying Motor Component
Broken doll: mends approximately (B)	Representational thought	Controlled arm and hand movements
Differentiates scribble from stroke (B)	Precise imitations	Developing crayon grasp and visual perceptual discrimination
Attempts to activate flashlight (E)	Causality	Fine motor control

E: Item from the Early Intervention Developmental Profile
B: Item from the Bayley Scales of Infant Development

Infant Play: A Reflection of Cognitive and Motor Development

Application to Assessment and Programming

Piaget's description of the stages of the sensorimotor period can be very useful in the assessment of infants with developmental disabilities. It provides a framework in which to analyze the cognitive components of developmental tasks, which, when combined with information on neuromotor and psychosocial development, provides a complete picture not only of *what* a child can do, but also *why* the child is doing it.

Observations of play through formal testing or informal sessions can be used to identify specific themes within a child's play. Children respond to toys in ways that express both their cognitive development and motor capabilities. The characteristics of these responses can be seen as a theme that recurs in a child's play regardless of the specific toy being used. From this theme, ideas about a child's skills can be generated.

A theme usually reflects a child's current and dominant play behaviors or schemas. The most common themes observed in evaluations and their corresponding cognitive stages are outlined below.

Theme	*Cognitive State*
Reaches, grasps, mouths toy	Primary Circular Reaction
Grasps, bangs, shakes, and mouths toy	Secondary Circular Reaction
Rotates toy in space while looking at it and pokes at parts before playing with toy	Coordination of Secondary Schemas
Attempts to do presented tasks but often takes apart pieces of puzzles or pegboards to replace parts or try a new piece in the space	Tertiary Circular Response
Performs tasks after a pause, as though thinking and planning a response	Invention of New Schemas Through Mental Combinations

Once a theme has been identified, the specifics of a child's play can be analyzed in terms of the development of the concepts of object constancy, spatiality, imitation, and causality, as well as an evaluation of the motor skills necessary to express these cognitive concepts. From this information, an understanding of a child's strengths and weaknesses can be derived.

For example, a child shown how to release a block into a container may respond by putting a hand into the container without releasing the block. Is the child demonstrating an imitation skill? Or is a demonstration of spatial concept hindered by a lack of voluntary release? The answer will determine whether the child needs to further develop a cognitive concept or a motor skill.

It is through the synthesis of information concerning cognitive, neuromotor, and psychosocial development that a real understanding of a child's play activities—or lack of them—can be derived.

This information is especially necessary when evaluating and treating infants and young children who are developmentally disabled and whose play may be correspondingly affected. It is important that the reasons behind a child's inability to perform a particular task be understood in order to develop the most effective treatment plan or educational objectives. Often such objectives are based on an observation of the child's highest developmental task and writing the next highest skill on the developmental checklist as an objective or goal. While this approach is acceptable, it falls short of taking into consideration a synthesis of information about neuromotor and cognitive development. It does not look at the underlying motor skill or the cognitive concept necessary for its performance. Nor does it correlate the reason behind a child's inability to perform the task with the information derived from the assessment.

To achieve this integration of assessment information and apply it to writing objectives, the following questions are helpful:

1. Is the infant's overall development delayed?

Assuming that the child is delayed enough to qualify for intervention services, it is helpful to look at the characteristics of the delay. If the child is at the same level in each area assessed (i.e., motor, cognitive, language), then the major problem is an overall delay similarly affecting all areas.

For effective intervention, goals should be written to facilitate the next-to-emerge concepts in cognitive development, as well as skills in other developmental areas. This will ensure that cognitive development and commensurate motor skills are mutually supportive. In addition, factors of developmental rate and etiology of the delay (environment vs. endogenous) should be used to ensure that goals address a child's unique needs.

2. Is the infant's expression of cognitive development being affected by delays or disorders in motor development?

Such a consideration is particularly applicable to children with neuromotor problems such as hypotonia, weakness, asymmetries, tremors, ataxic or athetoid movements, or spasticity. Such children may be attentive to an evaluation task and attempt its completion. Through task adaptations, proper positioning, and/or facilitation of appropriate muscle tone and movement, they may actually demonstrate their play abilities.

It is important that these children find ways to continue to facilitate cognitive development and allow for its expression in play despite underlying motor problems. It may be years, for example, before a child may demonstrate adequate head and neck control, but this should not prevent the development of the play-related concepts of object constancy, causality, spatiality, and imitation skills.

3. Does the infant demonstrate the variety of play skills characteristic of his or her developmental level?

A child may perform a variety of tasks typical of a particular developmental level, but a lack of quality and diversity may be present. This may be seen in such areas as the child's inability to attend to a task or perform only after much support and redirection. A child may demonstrate several play schemas, but they may seem too dominant and self-stimulating or perseverative. A child may also show a qualitative split in play skills; manipulation tasks, for example, may be performed at a much higher level than more abstract problem-solving tasks.

This information must also be utilized so that other necessary skills such as attention and the ability to change tasks are developed. Play behaviors that are developmentally appropriate may become self-stimulatory for a severely retarded child, and goals should be written to break such a cycle. Finally, the development of splinter skills should be recognized and other cognitive concepts receive attention in order to prevent gaps in cognitive development.

In summary, Piaget's theory of the sensorimotor period can be helpful to explain the cognitive dimensions of a child's play. With this information integrated into a knowledge of the child's neuromotor and psychosocial development, assessments can yield information that is more helpful in formulating effective developmental plans for infants and young children who are developmentally disabled.

References

1. Gruber H, Voneche, JJ: *The Essential Piaget: An Interpretive Reference and Guide*. New York: Basic Books, Inc., 1977
2. Flavell, J: *Cognitive Development*. Englewood Cliffs, NJ: Prentice-Hall, 1977
3. Richmond, PG: *An Introduction to Piaget*. New York: Basic Books, 1971
4. Ginsburg, H, Opper, S: *Piaget's Theory of Intellectual Development: An Introduction*. Englewood Cliffs, NJ: Prentice-Hall, 1969

Related Readings

Bayley, Nancy. *Bayley Scales of Infant Development*. New York: The Psychological Corporation, 1969.

Piaget, Jean. *The Origins of Intelligence in Children*. New York: International Universities Press, 1952.

Rogers, Sally, Donovan, Carol, et al: Early intervention developmental profile. In Schafer, D Sue and Moersch, Martha. *Developmental Programming for Infants and Young Children*. Ann Arbor: University of Michigan Press, 1981.